# Defragme

# So…

*John Sawkins*

**chipmunkapublishing**
the mental health publisher

Published by
Chipmunkapublishing
PO Box 6872
Brentwood
Essex CM13 1ZT
United Kingdom

**http://www.chipmunkapublishing.com**



Chipmunkapublishing gratefully acknowledge the support of Arts Council England.

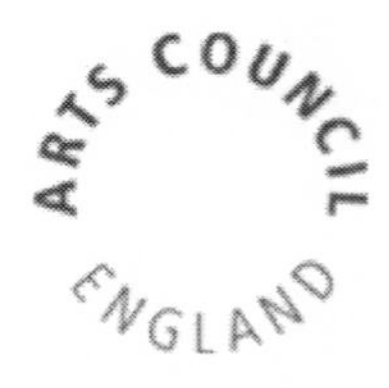

## Acknowledgements

The author would like to express his appreciation to everyone who has contributed to this book. In some cases, it will have been the experiences of friends and relations: without using these real-life stories as the basis for the subject matter, it would have been impossible to give a true picture of what 'reality' is like, both for mentally-ill patients, and for their carers and relations.

The author is likewise indebted to ideas espoused by professionals in the psychiatric and psychological fraternity – of both the mainstream and alternative varieties. It is hoped that some of these challenges to conventional thinking will generate new ways of looking at mental health altogether, with the inevitable ***questioning*** of existing remedies and anticipated outcomes that will need to take place.

The author extends particular gratitude to Aileen, Denise, Caroline, Stuart, Katrina and Maggie for exposing themselves to aberrant ways of thinking: the fact that they have emerged virtually unscathed is reassuring! He is also grateful for feedback from Ross White at the University of Glasgow, and from Lesley Berk at The University of Melbourne, Australia. Their recommendations have been taken on board, so I trust that the numerous redrafts will have eventually presented the reader with a more logical and cohesive structure than heretofore. Nevertheless, he makes no apologies for leaving much of the dialogue in its original version, primarily to preserve its authenticity. This is not by any means a ***novel***, in the conventional sense!

He extends his thanks to the artist, Professor Ian Scott, whose ideas about reclaiming identity seem to chime in somewhat with his own notion of the defragmentation process. The positive encouragement from Professor Ian Brown (formerly Drama Director at the Arts Council of England) has been instrumental in his decision to press ahead with this venture.

**Front cover design by Aileen Paton**

## John Sawkins (born 03.09.1948, Halifax, West Yorkshire): Recovery Story

Recovery tends to imply some notion of going back to your old self. After all, that is what your friends and relations would most like – perhaps clinicians, too. For the author, however, this was not to be an option. He decided to dump the garbage and start afresh with a new persona, after experiencing a hypo-manic episode just at the turn of the millennium.

Like many who experience the life-changing effects of having had a nervous break-down, he found himself impelled to cultivate a totally different existence to that of the person he used to be. Fortunately for him, his employers were sufficiently sympathetic to allow him to indulge his more creative side and he effectively abandoned the modern language teaching he had done for thirty years, lecturing instead in more creative pursuits such as music and photography.

That is not to say that he had never had such interests, however. It was just that he never found the time to indulge them. After the break-down (which, incidentally, he regards as being the start of a therapeutic healing process), he could sense the need to adopt more right-brain oriented thinking, and a number of long-cherished aspirations came to fruition as a result. He felt the need to remove the clutter from his thinking, jettison the unwanted baggage and embrace a fascinating - if somewhat more challenging - future.

First of all, he recorded a CD of songs he had written back in 1968. Then he joined the Caithness Big Band and tried to teach himself bass guitar – in that order! he subsequently joined the North Coast Jazz Band and has been with them for around eight years now. More recently, he succeeded in getting his poems ***Rare Frequencies*** published through Chipmunka.

Recovery has been achieved by following his own best instincts and reading widely about mental illness, the history of its treatment and opinions of a wide variety of professionals who have challenged the received wisdom of their colleagues particularly concerning the long-term use of medication to modify behaviour patterns.

Taking up advocacy work through Advocacy Highland proved to be a kind of therapy for the author. He needed to get out of the self-pitying self obsession that isolation can bring. It is important, he feels, to avoid scenarios where negative thoughts and downward spiral syndromes are reinforced.

So what was it, you may rightly ask, that he recovered ***from***? To be honest, he is not exactly sure, but since he exhibited some cyclothymic behaviour, that might have suggested bipolar just as the psychiatrist initially thought; but there were also other aspects of his behaviour patterns that did not quite fit the bill.

During the four weeks he spent in a psychiatric hospital, he had no choice but to take the medication (haloperidol, procycladine and zopiclone); but once he was out of there – and he is not necessarily implying that this was the most advisable course of action, though, at the time, it seemed quite reasonable – he decided to go cold turkey. Most folk who try this end up regretting it, for various reasons: some realise that they cannot function without their medication, and, however reluctantly, are forced to acknowledge ***the error of their ways***. Others find the detoxification process altogether too horrendous. Still, he decided to ride out the storm, and this took about four weeks. He has not taken any form of medication now for ten years since that date.

His employer did not wish him to return to work as quickly as he himself had hoped, so, in the interim, he needed to find something useful to do. He discovered ***The Stepping Stones***, a local drop-in facility for people with mental health issues, and soon found out that part of his therapy was to be found in acting as a volunteer. The advantage for the centre was that, having experienced a similar state of mind to the users of the centre (schizophrenia, bipolar, borderline personality disorder, etc), the author was better able to converse with them. Self-disclosure can do wonders when trying to open up people to discussion. He did poetry, art and music with the members and it was during such activities that spontaneous discussion arose. In helping others, he discovered an ability to help himself: his preoccupation with his condition and that destructive form of self-obsession that seems to accompany mental illness started to ebb away, as he found himself increasingly interested in and concerned about the issues preoccupying the members.

Six months after his "episode", he was pronounced sufficiently recovered to return to his former job as section leader for communications in a college of further education. It was to be a further four years before he took on additional work as a volunteer with Advocacy Highland. He would like to think that his contribution to tribunals, meetings, and care review plans has made a significant difference, in a positive way.

There appeared to be three choices facing him as the would-be recoverer: independence, dependency or interdependence. He preferred the latter, though he could see the attractions of the other two, as well. In some ways, he learned most from fellow-sufferers, and this is where his concept of interdependence started, but he instinctively knew that he would eventually have to learn to be interdependent in a world that did not solely comprise fellow-sufferers.

Medication and the various professional services, he feels, can inadvertently lead you down the road to dependency. This can encourage co-dependency issues, where both supporter and sufferer have difficulties weaning themselves off the relationship. Independence was another alternative, but, as he was soon to discover, ***no man is an island***, and we need our friends and partners in order to lead a half-way normal life. He puts his road to recovery down in no small measure to meeting his wife, Aileen, whom he married in 2006. Whether he has totally "recovered" is for others to judge, but at sixty-one he can say with some degree of certainty that he now very much enjoys life with all its little ups and downs.

John Sawkins, 18 December 2009.

## Prologue

***Defragmenting the Soul*** spent a whole life time in its gestation, though, in truth, the bulk of its planning came about during the nine years that followed the author's mental breakdown early in the auspicious year of 2000. The title emerged from a poem written by the author in August 2006 entitled ***Dis-integration***[1]. It had the equipotential to become a kind of self-help book, or, as will be detected in certain parts of the novel, an academic work – though the need for academic rigour and reputable references would, it is felt, have deprived the reader of several opportunities to suspend disbelief, and hence go along with many 'flights of fancy' in order to gain a better insight into the multidimensional facets of mental illness. For the poetic licence taken, the author offers no apologies. The author has never admitted to hearing voices, except when he was amongst [safe] friends. The latter were generally some way down the long journey to recovery, and keen to share their bizarre experiences, not with a psychiatrist who linked their 'symptoms' with one of the many learned articles he may have read at medical school, and who, himself, possibly may never (though the author has to concede that many psychiatrists have) personally experienced the above phenomena that generally resulted in the label 'schizophrenic' being appended to the patient; we needed our experiences affirmed, not challenged, and this we got from fellow-sufferers who had been there, done that and got the T-shirt. Our shared recollections of guardian angels and spirit guides reassured us that this was an all-too-common phenomenon, and not just a figment of our imagination, or a hallucination, no less. The author was gratified to discover that even atheists encountered such figures when they experienced mental illness. The author spent just four weeks in a psychiatric institution and that was enough to have driven him round the bend if he had not already been there. He had to take ***haloperidol*** under supervision, a drug at the time seen by the psychiatric profession as something of a panacea for bipolar / schizophrenia, (N.B. it **seems** often a case of ***one size fits all*** medication) but he discontinued its use, going 'cold turkey' immediately on his release from hospital (Don't try this at home, folks!). It came to his attention that one of the team who treated him had warned his wife to stay well clear of him in future, since he was a highly dangerous paranoid schizophrenic. If that truly had been the case, he must have been the only schizophrenic to have survived without need of any medication from the time he left hospital, nine years ago, without coming to the subsequent attention of the authorities. If, alternatively, he was, as previously indicated, bipolar, on the other hand, he was fortunate enough to enjoy equal good fortune in escaping sundry concoctions administered orally or by syringe under compulsory treatment orders. 'Good job the family did not decide to have

[1] Published by Chipmunkapublishing © John Sawkins 2008

him sectioned', he thought: as a 'voluntary' patient, his human rights were marginally better protected.

Medical staff, it must be said, behaved at all times in accordance with high ethical standards and clearly acted in what they perceived to be the best interests of the patients. With the advent of the internet, the medical arrogance of yesteryear has diminished somewhat, with staff now more willing to negotiate aspects of treatment, and genuinely sympathetic to the needs and plight of the individual, but sadly still dancing to the tune of the pharmaceutical industry.

**John Sawkins, July 3rd 2009**

## Introduction

Though the main character, Matthew, inevitably has many character traits in common with the author, he is really more of a ***composite*** mixture of a whole plethora of personalities, borderliners[2] and eccentrics, and acts as a mouthpiece for their shared plight, advocating on their behalf, too, at times. Since Matthew was never content to be just one ***in***dividual, he became what might consequently be referred to as a ***dividual***. We follow his various reincarnations, as he flits, like a butterfly, between professions, roles and identities. Though his character is by no means unsullied, (he's more of an anti-hero) he eventually finds redemption, after he agrees to dump his charade of an identity and become, instead, what he might have been.

The reader will be faced by a number of challenges from the very start, for which a paradigm shift in his or her ***Weltanschauung***[3] may be required. Characters interact and join discussions across past, present and future time zones, both face-to-face and through the use of virtual reality devices. The dead communicate with the living and vice versa. They do this by meeting up inside Matthew's head. Unless the reader has experienced a world where he or she can no longer differentiate between reality and fantasy, the blurring of the distinction between the two will be hard to imagine. Suffice it to say, that for some of ***us***, our fantasy world is altogether more vivid, exciting and 'real' than our shared 'reality' with you ***normal*** people!

Language plays a key role in Matthew's existence. He is constantly on the look-out for meaning. This perhaps justifies the inclusion of some rather esoteric material that flits from etymology to plays-on-words, occasionally across a number of foreign languages: primarily these are French, Latin and German. Just as he likes to extract meaning, however, Matthew is equally fascinated by the process of ***encryption*** of meaning. The roles he most successfully adopts are those of intermediary, and whether as a code-breaker, an interpreter or a medium, Matthew would no doubt have excelled, had he taken such opportunities offered to him when he was a young adult.

Like the communist German writer, Bertolt Brecht, Matthew has scant regard for religion, but he draws on the stories from the Bible in much the same way as Brecht did. And like Saint Paul, who 'saw the light' on the road to Damascus, Matthew, too, suddenly has his eyes opened after a lifetime of visual impairment, both literally and figuratively speaking. Whether we are believers or non-believers, there does appear to be an identifiable 'God spot' that occasionally lights up during functional

---

[2] Borderline Personality Disorder

[3] Philosophy (Way of looking at the world)

magnetic resonance imaging. (fMRI). Perhaps mankind needs to rely on leaps of faith from time to time to adjust the intellectual balance which tends to be always biased in favour of the so-called 'laws' of ***science***.

Along with the clutter of a superabundance of material possessions that really could do with recycling out to charity shops, and the like, Matthew has amassed during his lifetime a veritable dung-heap of emotional baggage and intellectual ***crap***. Jean-Paul, the spirit-guide, assists him in the process of exorcising his demons, thus making space for new ideas and plans. In the bewildered state we find Matthew, the figure of Jean-Paul emerges as a trustworthy beacon who can guide him back towards sanity. Matthew has to decide what is truly worth keeping, valuable and collectable; what needs to be recycled; and what needs to go for garbage disposal. But he does not automatically throw things away: he first has to see if they can be fixed or repaired; just like the broken souls of the mentally ill. We all have a duty to do everything in our power to help them recover and not effectively consign them to the 'happy dumping ground'.

Matthew was highly sceptical of scientists' claims to have recently identified the genes responsible for schizophrenia: tiny genetic mutations known as ***single nucleotide polymorphisms***. Since the same research no longer made a distinction between bipolar and schizophrenia, he promptly contacted Catherine and Alison, Brian and Graham to inform them that he was not so different from them, after all. Bipolars are perhaps no more and no less dysfunctional than schizophrenics: they have just been given a different badge to wear. So what does this ground-breaking research all mean? For the sufferers, remarkably little. It signifies merely that yet another generation of drugs will be manufactured for compliant zombies to take, just in order to make money for the shareholders in the pharmaceuticals industry.

The drugs, according to Matthew, were never administered for the ultimate benefit of the patient: they are just one more weapon in the armoury of control by the state that sees sedation of the individual as the safest option for the rest of society. It encourages families and friends to collude in this myth that 'he/she will only get better if he/she takes his/her medication'. In reality, it is a case of if you are ***out of mind*** we would prefer you to be ***out of sight,*** locked away for as long as it takes. Medication suits the family, the community, society: it rarely suits the individual. It is just more convenient for the other 75% of you that the 25% minority, takes its punishment like a man, or more accurately, from a statistical point of view, ***like a woman***. (Could it be that males are more inclined to opt out of health services because they are by nature less trusting of medicine, and not because they are stupid, as some health campaigns would have us believe?)

**Operis personae**

| | |
|---|---|
| 1. | Alan (a socialist colleague) |
| 2. | Alice (Matthew's confidante) |
| 3. | Andrea (a journalist) |
| 4. | Andy (a forensic detective) |
| 5. | Anita (Matthew's wife) |
| 6. | Arthur (Matthew's father ) |
| 7. | Belinda (a fellow-student) |
| 8. | Bert (Matthew's boss) |
| 9. | Brian (a schizophrenic friend) |
| 10. | Burkhart (a German industrialist) |
| 11. | Carol (a friend of Matthew's) |
| 12. | Cassandra (a new age shopkeeper) |
| 13. | Charon (the ferryman) |
| 14. | Connie (a German teenager) |
| 15. | Dave (Matthew's room-mate in the psychiatric hospital) |
| 16. | Dee (a sociologist) |
| 17. | Dieter (a German revolutionary) |
| 18. | Donnie (an audio technician) |
| 19. | Doris (Matthew's Fräulein) |
| 20. | Dr Martin (Matthew's G.P.) |
| 21. | Dr Sanderson (an optician) |
| 22. | Dr Scott (a Scottish psychiatrist) |
| 23. | Edna (Matthew's mother) |
| 24. | Elaine (Matthew's barrister) |
| 25. | Eleanor (Matthew's granddaughter) |
| 26. | Eric (a film director) |
| 27. | Eve (Matthew's seductress) |
| 28. | Frank (a priest) |
| 29. | Gary (Matthew's childhood friend) |
| 30. | George (an undertaker) |
| 31. | Gilbert (a psychiatrist's son) |
| 32. | Godfrey (a computer whizz-kid) |
| 33. | Graham (a schizophrenic friend) |
| 34. | Hans (the son of a rich German industrialist) |
| 35. | Hazel (a personnel manager) |
| 36. | Helene (a colleague of Matthew's) |
| 37. | Honey (Matthew's mistress) |
| 38. | Iain (a psychiatric nurse) |
| 39. | Ian (a dramatist) |
| 40. | Ivan (Matthew's imaginary enemy) |
| 41. | Jean-Paul (Matthew's spiritual guide) |
| 42. | Jim (an American colleague) |

| 43. Jimmy (an inspiring colleague) |
| --- |
| 44. John "Mr Messy" (an artist) |
| 45. Johnny (a writer) |
| 46. Jonathan (a critic) |
| 47. Kate (Matthew's daughter) |
| 48. Kenny (Matthew's friend) |
| 49. Ken (a soldier) |
| 50. Leonard (a tour-guide in Cuba) |
| 51. Les (an acoustics engineer) |
| 52. Liam (a prisoner) |
| 53. "Little Brother" an unnamed individual [paranoia] |
| 54. Liz (Matthew's cousin) |
| 55. Luke (Matthew's grandson) |
| 56. Marjorie (Matthew's protégée) |
| 57. Mark (Matthew's son) |
| 58. Matthew |
| 59. Mavis (a medium) |
| 60. Mick (a taxi-driver) |
| 61. Mike (a famous folk musician) |
| 62. Moira (Matthew's work colleague) |
| 63. Mrs Feather (Matthew's head teacher in primary school) |
| 64. Niall (a retired doctor) |
| 65. Paul "Vladimir" (A stand-up comedian) |
| 66. Paolo (a media-man) |
| 67. Persephone (a midwife) |
| 68. Peter (a pianist) |
| 69. Pete (a builder) |
| 70. Rich (a Viet Nam War Veteran) |
| 71. Ricky (a sceptical scientist) |
| 72. Roy (a Conservative councillor) |
| 73. Sheila (an NLP enthusiast) |
| 74. Sean (Matthew's mentor) |
| 75. Simon (an agoraphobic) |
| 76. Sirian (a famous Scottish artist) |
| 77. Steve (an accountant) |
| 78. Dr Süss "Suggs" (an English psychiatrist) |
| 79. Sylvia (Matthew's girlfriend at college) |
| 80. Theodora (Matthew's work-colleague) |
| 81. Veronica (a librarian and archivist) |
| 82. Volker (a German student) |
| 83. Wolfgang (A German revolutionary) |
| 84. Yorick (A Highland Poet) |

The characters and events in this story are purely fictional. If, in describing the alleged behaviour of psychiatrists, politicians, teachers, journalists, writers, family members, ***et al.*** any similarities with real-life situations should become apparent, this is neither intentional nor accidental, on the author's part, but practically inevitable.[4]

[4] The author is indebted for the above [abridged] caveat to Heinrich Böll's preface in his book, ***The Lost Honour of Katharina Blum.***

# *Episode I*

## Chapter One – The square peg

**"The curious paradox is that when I accept myself just as I am, then I can change."**
**Carl Rogers**

In Matthew's day, perseverance was deemed to be a great virtue. It was for this reason – as well as the necessity of earning a living – that Matthew stuck with a job for life, namely that of the teacher.

Numerologically speaking, Matthew was a 'seven'. This meant that he had many admirable positive qualities, but equally, he had some horrific negative personality traits. He was consequently blessed with the gifts of wisdom, resilience, perspicacity and meditation; but cursed with hypercriticism, inaction, unsociability and morbidness. His determination, a positive quality, could at any time swing over into bloody-mindedness, clearly a negative trait of character. His frenetic cerebral activity burned up the calories at a rate of knots, and when combined with the inevitable adrenalin rush, it produced a high metabolic rate which in turn ensured that he rarely in his life put on any weight.

As a consequence, Matthew had a gaunt appearance, almost emaciated, in fact. For most of his adult life he hid behind a full beard, and sported oversized spectacles. He found it hard to maintain eye-contact, particularly when his interlocutors had the eyes of a predator, rather than those of a gazelle. He never looked what you might call ***relaxed***, appearing, instead, to clench his teeth and fists whenever he became agitated. Rather than use his hands to enhance his delivery of communication, he always seemed awkward with them, not knowing whether to fold his arms in a defensive gesture, put his hands in his pockets (which seemed rude) or place them on his hips (which affected a vaguely camp attitude). His face was dead pan – no obvious expression whatsoever. All this accounts, along with his aversion to outdoor pursuits, such as football, for the virtual absence of any wrinkles across his forehead in middle age.

Through the mask, Matthew did his utmost to ***sound through***, as the ***persona***[5] required. Which character would emerge today? So many options; so many possibilities. Would he go for the crowd-pleaser and bask in the adulation of his disciples or would he for once risk alienating them by offering them a glimpse of his true self?

"Matthew! Wake up!" shouted Sue, his talking-therapist. This was all part of Matthew's rehabilitation. Matthew attended weekly psychotherapy

---

[5] The meaning of words will be a crucial factor in Matthew's analysis of his predicament

sessions during the spring of 2000 at a clinic situated to the south of Manchester. Sue was the kind of therapist Matthew felt he could warm to, because she exhibited the same kind of racing thoughts as himself in her communication with others. He liked the way her mind worked, flitting from one topic to the next almost effortlessly, but unlike his own mind, Sue's pursued a much clearer logical process. She was young, slim, and quite petite. She had penetrating eyes that did not allow your mind to wander too far, before you were dragged back to Earth with a jolt. For a mere butterfly like himself, it was as though Sue were the lepidopterist sticking her pins into her client to stop him flitting from one topic to the next, in dilettante fashion.

"You were about to tell me how you ended up becoming a teacher, despite your obvious aversion to that profession," said Sue.
"Teaching is rather like acting, though it differs from acting in the sense that you have to put on a variety of shows for a number of audiences up to thirty times a week," said Matthew. "Completing my teaching practice in Ponders End, Enfield - where my college tutor claimed to have had a nervous breakdown - was a real baptism of fire. 'Do you want to try me on?' challenged a sturdily-built skinhead of the day, thumbs tucked menacingly behind his braces. Needless to say, I resisted the temptation to rise to the challenge, and respectfully declined the boy's invitation to do battle."

"Like most teachers, Matthew, you've still got a lot to learn," said Sue. "You're always telling everybody else how to run their lives."
"I'm a bit like Bertolt Brecht in that respect," said Matthew.
"Yes, but you're constantly firing out didactic messages, believing that you can get people to see the error of their ways by hectoring them and telling them that only you could possibly know what is best for them. Instead, you could say, 'Look, this is how I deal with depression: it might only work for me, but I'm sharing it with you just in case my strategies could work for you. Even though I personally am vehemently ***anti*** prescription drugs, I realise they represent for some people their salvation – just as for others their salvation might be religion."

"Do you realise," said Sue, "how often you play the dictator?" Matthew apologised, "Please bear with me: it is part of my personality." Sue smiled, "Perhaps you were quite suited to teaching after all. After all, bossiness is a trait commonly found in teachers. I'd hazard a guess that you might have gravitated towards teaching because, subconsciously, you were looking for more control over your life." Matthew was about to reflect on that thought, when Sue interrupted his reveries with the next item on her tick-list. "Let's turn to your childhood influences," said Sue, "How did you get on with your school-mates?"

recruits how the team without a leader failed to negotiate the assault course successfully, whilst the team with an externally imposed leader (presumably selected for his leadership skills) all made it across the river in one piece. Needless to say, Matthew elected not to pursue this career any further, determined to prove that the leader does not necessarily have to be ***der Führer***.

He once saw an excellent cartoon drawing, highlighting the absolute plethora of management styles. Round the table sat such recognisable stereotypes as the little Hitler, identified here by the fact that he was wearing a Napoleon hat; the two-headed leader with one comment to your face and another behind your back; the clown, who is just about tolerated because he is quite amusing, however ineffective he is at his job: most of the images, it must be said, were rather uncomplimentary caricatures of leaders in general. Matthew realised that he had been assuming on a daily basis as many as twelve different leadership styles, and felt that such inconsistency must surely have been confusing to ***the troops***.

However, the one advantage of being in this management position was that he was allowed to try out some of his off-the-wall ideas with the tacit blessing of his superiors. Simply by looking at his signature, any graphologist worth his salt could have seen that Matthew was an (unconventional) ideas man. He had insisted from his early school years in writing the letter 'S' back-to-front, despite persistent attempts from his teachers to discourage this. Over the years, his scrawl had become practically illegible, even to himself! The surname petered out, indicating perhaps that he could come up with the ideas and maybe get them off the ground, but thereafter he became bored and wanted to busy himself with another potential project. He left such minutiae to Peter, ***the completer***.

## Chapter two – the outsider

**Sometimes I'm happy, sometimes I'm sad.**
**Things are good or things are bad.**
**Can't make it now, the past's too late,**
**And tomorrow is too long to wait.**

**(JS/1968)**

Matthew had always felt different in some way from the other kids. He preferred to observe rather than participate. Where other kids would clearly enjoy diving into the swimming pool in the summer or having a snowball-fight in the winter, Matthew would say, 'I think I'll just watch.' Even as an adult, this tendency did not entirely desert him. It was as though he felt undeserving of such uninhibited licence. Indeed, Anita could frequently be heard remonstrating with him over his puritanical streak. He seemed to have no vices, but what was worse was that he could hardly disguise his disdain for the overindulgence of his guests. He made a big point of it one evening, when Anita had asked some friends round for drinks. He pointedly refused to engage in a communal glass of wine, opting for fruit juice, that evening. This clearly had its effect on the guests who felt obliged to restrict their consumption for the evening to one glass of wine each.

It was as though Matthew was deliberately doing everything in his power to set himself apart from the rest of society. He was complicit in reinforcing his ***outsider*** status and was not prepared to make even minimal compromises with a view to becoming accepted. Though he understood all the psychological tricks that could be used to ingratiate himself with the group, he generally opted to alienate everyone by deliberately disagreeing with them. In a way, it was an intellectual game. What he was effectively saying was, 'I don't necessarily hold an opposing view to you, but if I take the role of devil's advocate, I can still win the argument hands down.'

In a drama lesson, Matthew had once repeated the experiment where one student is sent out of the room and the remaining group members are told to close ranks with the express purpose of excluding that student. The teacher then meets separately with the student, encouraging him/her to try everything in the book to get himself (or herself) accepted. If the individual shows sufficient charm or appeals to the others' sense of fair play, etc., he/she usually manages to overcome the artificial social barriers the teacher has created.

Matthew had also learned a great deal about the use of body language. Face-to-face could often be very confrontational, whilst turning your back on someone sent out the message loud and clear that you did not wish to communicate with them. He knew from neuro-linguistic programming (NLP), that mirroring was a very powerful tool. Sometimes, just to prove its effectiveness, he would mimic the body language of his interlocutors and see them warm to his ideas. He extended this to his choice of vocabulary and turns of phrase, noting that each individual, (as well as speaking in their local geographical dialect and their own sociolect which perhaps differed according to the company they were in), used their own favourite words and phrases (their idiolect). As we will see, Matthew had previously used this knowledge to help in his espionage activities. The chosen target would subconsciously feel flattered that they had found someone who ***spoke the same language*** as themselves, but was blissfully unaware of the subterfuge that had been perpetrated upon them. Obviously, Matthew enjoyed the power that this awareness gave him over others. Rather amusingly, he met his match in Sheila, who recognised what was going on just as she was attempting to pull the same trick on him. At that point, they both burst out laughing, having to acknowledge their mutual indebtedness to neuro-linguistic programming.

Matthew had a distinct persecution complex and seemed to always sense people were coming up behind him or talking about him. (This ticked the box – in his psychiatrist's checklist – for paranoid tendencies). It was very much for this reason that you would rarely find him at the centre of things. At parties, he would ensure that his back was to the wall, and that he had a clear view of people entering and leaving the room. Jean-Paul, his spirit guide, was to teach him the wisdom of not having his back to the door if he shared an office; he also recommended proximity to a window and Matthew tried in future to negotiate such a location, wherever possible.

Matthew was not always anti-social: indeed, if the mood took him, he could be the life and soul of the party. (The psychiatrist ticked the box that indicated 'bipolar'). This was rather hit-and-miss, however. It depended where he was on his bipolar cycle. This possibly needs further elaboration. Matthew was reminded by Brian, who himself was schizophrenic, how lucky manic-depressives are in comparison to schizophrenics. "You can actually function quite well in society. You can dispatch mountains of work when you're manic, you can be a real asset to your employer." Matthew looked back on the colossal feats he had performed in his manic phases: he had produced his Master's thesis at the same time as teaching and working the taxis in Manchester in 1981. Sleep had been an extravagance that he dismissed as an unnecessary indulgence. He sometimes used these brief spells of abundant energy to complete the likes of decorating jobs around the house.

It was the inconsistency, however, that neither Anita, nor especially his children, could comprehend. Children need parenting to be consistent. It does not matter that much if parenting is authoritarian or laissez-faire, but when it swings from one extreme to the other, the kids really do not know where they stand. One minute, Matthew would be full of beans, alert and productive, the next, he would be dosing off on the sofa, with his head on the cushions, oblivious of what time of day it might be.

In retrospect, it was clear that Matthew needed to compensate for these immense bursts of energy that sometimes lasted for days. In order to gain more control over these phases, Matthew decided to keep a diary where he could plot the high points and low points. What might for the average person seem to be predictable highs would be the holidays. With Matthew, however, this was far from the case. His cycle generally encompassed a period of twelve weeks, with Christmas, Easter and the start of summer holidays coinciding with his absolute nadirs. It was a kind of endogenous depression, totally unaffected by whatever positive events were happening in his life at the time. The start of the new school year was a similar low-point. Midway between these points, Matthew was always at his most productive. He had met others with the bipolar condition whose cycle was much shorter: sometimes the mood would fluctuate within a matter of hours, or even minutes, so their ability to function effectively at work was seriously impeded.

Matthew began to realise why he had always avoided letting go and enjoying himself. It was because he knew that after the high followed the inevitable low, and by living life on a humdrum, mundane level, he thought he could escape the extremes. He would look forward to holidays and try to look back on them with fond nostalgia, but he could never totally immerse himself in the moment of that holiday – he always held some energy in reserve, and curiously, seemed to be in a world of his own, unrelated to the exciting events he should have been experiencing at the time. It was as though he inhabited some kind of parallel universe and was having to share his presence with simultaneous experiences elsewhere. His ***alter ego*** made regular trips into the domain co-inhabited by his spirit guide, Jean-Paul.

Later on in his life - more precisely in his 'other' life - Matthew did make a conscious effort to integrate and benefited greatly from the experience, finding himself invited to join organisations, clubs and bands. This paradoxically only happened, however, once he decided to stop trying to act out what he thought others expected of him. As soon as he dropped the various personae that he had adopted to suit different audiences, people started to accept him for who he was. For once in his life, he was able to play himself, and his essentially warm personality started to flourish for the first time ever. After wearing a mask for most of his life, he was suddenly able to revert to what was the essential Matthew.

Matthew very rarely practiced what he preached, reminding his disciples to 'do as I say, not as I do!' He urged them to enjoy the moment, whilst personally flitting, as many bipolar patients do, between fondness for a mythical golden age in the past and fear about an uncertain future. However, he would look forward to holidays, yet when they arrived, he was ***elsewhere***; not participating in the fun at all. Perhaps he was already there in the future, living out his life in some parallel universe.

## Chapter three – the seer

Looking back at his life, Matthew realised how prescient his song-writing had been in anticipating future events in his life. The songs had a prophetic dimension, with the young man warning the old man about missed opportunities:

***He contemplates his life while he's still young:***
***No mountain has he climbed, no song he's sung.***

The same song hints at the location of the Akashic records, too:

***The purpose of his life – he can't say why:***
***It's hidden in the secrets of the sky.***

***"Steps of Time"*** JS/1969

His detention in the psychiatric hospital had been similarly anticipated:

***I never could see, why they left reality***
***Till I too was standing by the stream***

***"Standing by the stream"*** JS/1971

As a child, Matthew had shown potential. He was grudgingly prepared to acknowledge that genetics was responsible for whatever creative talent he might have possessed. His maternal grandmother had been a well-known artist in the neighbourhood of Leicester. The oil painting entitled ***Chrysanthemums*** now hangs in the hall of his house. It had been painted way back in 1896. Rosa had also been a piano teacher and he attributed his own interest in music mainly to this inherited trait, though he also credited his father as having had - from the point of view of nurture - a more direct influence through his harmonica playing on cold winter nights. Arthur had noted Matthew's artistic skills whilst the latter was still at primary school and put his son down for a place at technical school with a view to him training to be a draftsman. Sadly, this was not to be. Matthew surprised many in passing the eleven plus exam and ending up in the A-stream of the local grammar school, where a whole new set of future options presented themselves to him.

Grammar was indeed one of the things Matthew mastered quite quickly and this accompanied a penchant for linguistics. However, it was the concept of time that fascinated him most, epitomised by the notion of a tense called the ***future-in-the-past continuous***. Thirty years on from his song-writing days, the enigmatic expressions contained within them now began to make sense.

The notion of the "overlapping steps of time" brought home to him the sheer artificiality of time with its convenient sub-divisions into past present and future. "Carpe diem" (seize the day) seemed always to be the best maxim for enjoying life.

Where had all this material come from? He did not feel like an imitator, or one who was simply a medium for dead poets:

> ***And who can doubt sincerity in our own thoughts?***
> ***Are we just vehicles to convey cheap reports?***

He recalled the notion of automatic writing and was fascinated by Rosemary Brown, the medium, who claimed to commune with the great musical composers to generate ***magna opera*** in their style. The one time he had cleared his head and simply allowed the pen to flow, the following bizarre set of lines had appeared:

> ***Their bones drum in time to a soft violin***
> ***That lures you in laughter, preserved in a grin.***
> ***Your will starts to weaken, you cannot resist,***
> ***In front of your eyes is a welcoming fist.***

To date their significance has not been revealed to him.

He envied people who were capable of phenomenological interaction, but felt pathologically attracted to the role of observer, rather than that of participant. The here and now escaped him – answers to two of the barrage of questions he would face during the interrogation from Jean-Paul, his spirit-guide, which was to challenge his ***Weltanschauung*** thirty years on.

Matthew thought forward (or was it backwards?) to the self-fulfilling prophesy that his 1970's song would produce:

> ***I often wondered who was standing, alone, beside the stream***
> ***I lacked that certain understanding for people in a dream.***

The fascination with a world of fantasy that once could only be dreamed of eventually led to total emersion in it, as a living heaven or a living hell. Luckily for Matthew, it was closer to the former than the latter, but, like any novel experience, it was not devoid of scary moments when he wondered if he would be able to distinguish fantasy from reality ever again.

Even back in 1971, whilst still a student, living in London, Matthew had secretly rather envied the world of schizophrenia. His strict religious upbringing had provided an extensive exposure to the Bible and the idea of ***speaking in tongues***. Even his rapacious consumption of foreign languages might be shown to have been initiated by biblical etymological references. The voice of Jean-Paul, his spirit guide, was – despite the traumatic experience accompanying it – a very reassuring voice. Strange though it may seem, the instructions from Jean-Paul were very rational. Sue had pointed out that any number of totally ludicrous instructions from voices can seem perfectly logical and reasonable to a poor deluded soul, but Jean-Paul seemed to provide the only exit strategy for Matthew from this nightmare of a twilight existence.

Matthew had always been a cerebral kind of individual. In fact, he almost took a pride in not expressing his emotions. So when he finally broke, all the emotional elements came gushing out uncontrollably. Looking back at his phone bill from that time, spookily coinciding with the turn of the millennium, he realised that he had spent hours conducting one-way conversations with his wife. Prior to that time, he had been virtually monosyllabic in his dialogue on the phone.

He much preferred the structure of English, an analytical language, to German, a synthetic language. Yet he could sense that his left brain was shutting down from overuse. It had served him well over the years where his job had required an analytical mind, but now it was time for the right brain to take over. How different the world seemed without the censoring filter of the left brain that used to direct his thinking! How refreshing it was to go with the gut reaction instead of agonising over the pros, cons and consequences!

Now, this right/left split had always preoccupied him. During the period when Matthew discovered that he had an intuitive ability for graphology, he had noted that handwriting tended to slant to the left in individuals more inclined to focus on past events, whilst those planning for the future would generally prefer a right slant. Matthew had also dabbled in palmistry, noting that the left hand showed the blueprint of what you could potentially achieve, whilst the right hand demonstrated the extent to which it had been realised.

Did this dichotomy also extend to so-called right / left-wing political thinking, he wondered? After all, he had been a socialist with certain liberal tendencies for most of his life, and yet here he was, standing in the ballot box, putting his cross against the name of the conservative candidate! Remarkable changes in perception were indeed occurring. Was he actually literally ***seeing*** the world differently from before? He even found himself lifting his cherished pint with his left hand, for a change.

The upshot of Matthew taking up drums – as opposed to guitar – the previous evening was quite bizarre. After practice, the band had all moved on to the local hostelry and Matthew had consumed his customary two pints

of ***Guinness***. It was not until the following morning that he experienced it. Peering back at him from the bathroom mirror were ***three*** eyes! He blinked. Then he looked up and down. Then he looked to the right and to the left. To give the reader an idea of ***what*** Matthew was seeing, you have to imagine what it was like for him when crossing the road, or climbing stairs. In the former case, looking right, he would see two images of the advancing traffic; looking to the left, the customary one image. In the latter example, the stairs morphed into a jumble of zigzag lines. He decided to get his vision checked by a professional. "How many fingers?" asked Dr Sanderson, the optician. Matthew smiled.
"I expected an optician, not a midwife," said Matthew. The optician ignored the comment, but as if to reinforce the confusion, began to induce ***dilation***, as he released drops of atropine into Matthew's eyes. In his discussions with the consultant, it seemed impossible to "identify the phantom", as requested.
"If I look to the left," said Matthew, "I see only the one finger pointing upwards. However, if I look to the right, I see two."
"I suppose you'll be having me believe you have three eyes next?" said the optician. "Well," said Matthew, "and what if I have?" (Mystics will recognise the significance of the third eye).

***Red and green must never be seen***, but Matthew clearly saw the optician's green and red circles, one *above* the other. As far as he could remember – and his previous eye test was a long time ago – the circles used to appear side by side. For six weeks, he had the luxury of two views of the world: as he looked down the road snaking off into the distance, he could see an image tinged with pink, and he much preferred this to its twin with the greenish hue. Unfortunately, he could not choose between them. Both images were there simultaneously.

He eventually succeeded in using ***Corel Draw*** to import two identical photographs superimposed one on top of the other. Taking great pains to keep the two images aligned at the left-hand side of the page, he selected the 'rotate' facility and moved the top image round by an angle of five degrees.
"There you are, that's what I am seeing," he said, plonking it down triumphantly on the optician's desk. A diagnosis of mini-stroke followed with ***mid-line shift*** as a partial explanation of the diplopia phenomenon. Matthew was relieved and gratified to eventually have his variant of double vision confirmed by the optician. He had the distinct impression that a hospital consultant would not have believed him, or had even thought he might be hallucinating, given his psychiatric history.

"Grains of sand," said Matthew, excitedly, "I can actually see microscopic specks of dust without descending to my hands and knees." When his eyesight returned to normal, he was pleasantly surprised to find that the

myopia for which he had worn corrective spectacles for most of his adult life had disappeared.
"You're legal to drive now, without glasses," confirmed the optician.

Matthew had gradually got used to restricted vision over time, so now a whole new world opened up where he could see people's faces. Friends were somewhat disconcerted by the new Matthew, who greeted them by name as he recognised them from the other side of the street. In the past, they had taken his apparent non-recognition of them to be aloofness, rudeness or just plain shyness. He felt like an old work-horse, retired from a life of drudgery and afforded the luxury of green pastures, once the blinkers were removed from his eyes. But the 'Tennessee Stud' was not yet ready for the knackers' yard. He started to feast his eyes on the young fillies, who had existed as a vision he could have only imagined in the past. Matthew's fascination, however, was not simply restricted to women. He was struck by the beauty of the landscapes, which now stood out in vivid detail. It made him want to evangelise, encouraging others to appreciate the pulchritudinous world we all share.

Though Matthew undoubtedly possessed considerable intellect and had now begun to learn how to handle his emotional intelligence, one more dimension was still to be explored: the spiritual dimension.

## Chapter four – the priest

Religion can be the salvation for some mentally ill patients: for others, however, it can equally well precipitate their downfall into insanity, as Matthew was to discover from some fellow-patients in the psychiatric ward. But for Matthew himself, this was not to be the case. He quickly realised that to save his soul, he desperately needed to regain the spiritual dimension to his life. The route to redemption seemed to come via Saint Paul, or was it perhaps Jean-Paul?

To truly become a real person, Matthew needed to retrieve his soul. Up until the point when he reached his mid-teens, he had been a devout worshipper, even, as a server, assisting the vicar with Holy Eucharist, but he had felt that need to escape the accompanying propaganda with its underlying Conservative message, partly because he felt this interpretation of the biblical texts undermined his working class origins. For example, he recalls one Sunday evening in Lightcliffe, when the Reverend White used the parable of the talents to demonstrate the virtues of capitalism: money needed to be invested wisely to gain a good return on one's investments – simply hiding your cash in the ground was foolish. Since Matthew had wanted to understand how this could possibly have squared with Christ's teachings, he decided to explore the analogy and to trace the etymology of the word 'talent'[7]. Matthew preferred to believe that the story was merely an analogy: he should exploit the God-given talents that he possessed, rather than waste his life on some job he detested just for its pecuniary advantage.

There had been a recurring character throughout his life and he attempted to make sense of the frequent encounters. Statistically, there are many people called Paul, and he could probably have read as many coincidences into encounters with Peter. Nevertheless, he felt some deep and significant connection with the name, Paul. On first attending primary school, he had formed a close relationship with a boy named Paul, only to experience the lad being taken away by his family to live in some distant part of the country, never to be seen again.

---

[7] It is true that, taking the expression literally, a talent (from the Greek τάλαντον ) had been a coin, like the Thaler, or more recently, the dollar, hence a monetary interpretation might follow. However, the ***figurative*** use of the word as we use it today is attributed to Matthew xxv 14-30.

At the age of eleven, the Reverend White had deemed Matthew capable of reading one of the lessons at the Christmas service. The text was guaranteed to have a lasting impression on him because it was taken from Saint Paul to the Corinthians.[8] When he won the prize for divinity – as the subject was then called – Matthew was presented with a book about Paul of Tarsus, and he was later to reflect on Saul's epiphany when he too began to see the world through different eyes. Even when he looked into his genealogy, Matthew found out that one derivation of his family name linked him with the relatives of Saul.

Even in his current semi-agnostic state, he liked the solace of churches. He now missed the sense of community that belonging to a church can offer. What could replace that ***place of safety***? The psychiatrists had usurped the role that the clergy used to perform, turning the concept of sanctuary into that of containment. Yet he could not acknowledge ever having signed his soul over to the devil at any point. It felt far more as if he had voluntarily relinquished little slithers of himself every time he felt obliged to compromise to fit in with others' expectations of him. The sad irony was that each successful modification to his personality once achieved failed to satisfy those demanding it. As soon as he effected the change they seemed to require, they moved the goal posts. In the process he felt he had surrendered another part of himself, or had the devil stolen it? His soul had gradually begun to fragment.

---

[8] Chapter XIII 1-13 ***And now abideth faith, hope and charity, but the greatest of these is charity.***

## Chapter five – the thief

Theft has acquired a whole new meaning in this digital age, but when Matthew was growing up, the difference between right and wrong in the acquisition of property was slightly less ambiguous. In 1955, when Matthew was at primary school in the West Riding of Yorkshire, his peer group had persuaded him to accompany them on a raid of the school orchard. Even at that age, he knew it was wrong, but it seemed like a victimless crime, since the apples were never harvested and would have been left to rot, in any case. The following day at school, Mrs Feather, the Headmistress, interrogated two likely lads who promptly confessed, though not before incriminating the other marginally less culpable kids who had really just gone along for the ride. She was shocked to find Matthew implicated, and expressed to him her disappointment that he had not come forward voluntarily before being fingered.

"You know the story from the bible about the Garden of Eden, don't you Matthew?" she said. "Stealing apples is like trying to steal knowledge. You have to earn the right to knowledge. If you want apples, you have to earn money to buy them, but with knowledge, it's different. In America, I hear you can buy degrees, but even so, you can't buy knowledge. I shall be keeping a close watch on you from now on, because I believe you can win your laurels, but that will certainly not happen if you come off the rails." The reader may wonder at the language used by the teacher to talk to a seven-year-old, but that was how it was in Matthew's day: teachers did not go out of their way to explain things in terms a child might comprehend. Consequently, Matthew retained the information, but only gradually began to understand its momentousness as he got older.

When he reached the appropriate stage identified by Piaget, he grasped the symbolic significance of the apple, as well as the fact that knowledge could be put to multifarious purposes; nefarious as well as admirable ones. 'Winning his laurels' began to make sense, once he started to study Latin, and 'coming off the rails' was to figure in his sociological study of adolescents. As for buying degrees, that service appears to have become a recent American import into this country.

In his time, Matthew had been the victim of burglary and knew how invasive that felt, but he had never intentionally stolen from anyone. Sundry books belonging to former friends he had never returned, though, to be fair, his friends had kept many of his, too; the same went for gramophone records. But he felt quite strongly about copyright. Since he had never got round to copyrighting the musical scores he had composed, it was no real surprise to him, when he discovered that someone he had once worked with had decided to capitalise on this fact. Matthew did not really mind his work being taken over in this way: in a sense, it was quite a compliment to its quality, but he personally just would not have felt good about palming someone else's work off as his own.

"Of course we comply with copyright law," said Tom. "We always pay the photographer, composer, playwright, writer, etc, whenever we use their original materials." But Matthew knew otherwise.
"I've seen the so-called 'creatives' nicking someone else's photo from the internet, then flipping it or otherwise modifying it, so it can't be traced back to the person who took the photo. Just about everyone has a printer at home that does photocopies. Who knows how many copies are taken of books and plays without paying royalties? Composers, on the other hand, have had to get more wiley. They eschew A4 as a precaution, hoping that this will deter pirates from trying to copy irregular formats. But performers lose out: CD's and DVD's are so easy to copy on the average computer, the Performing Rights Society is on a hiding to nothing most of the time."

"Where do you stand on the issue of intellectual property rights?" asked Anita, who had had some of her self-penned teaching ideas purloined by a rival college. "I was incensed that all the time and effort I had put into preparing open learning materials was taken advantage of in that way. Imagine picking up a copy of a commercially produced course to find your words staring back at you, verbatim!" Mathew agreed that this was an unacceptable state of affairs,
"How did the other college get a copy?" Anita was not sure,
"It may have been one of the students that passed it on, but I suspect it might even have been an unscrupulous colleague." Matthew considered the legal implications, "Couldn't you have sued, or demanded a cut of the revenue from the books?" Anita shook her head,
"whatever I generated in my role as a tutor would automatically have belonged to the college I was working for at the time," said Anita.
"Well, I think at least the college should have been reimbursed," said Matthew.

"And identity theft," said Matthew, "has that ever happened to you?" Anita shook her head, again, explaining why she thought it less likely in her case,
"There only appear to be two other individuals with the same surname as me. Even before the opportunity to Google my name, I used to check out sundry telephone directories for a Doppelgänger, but none appeared. Even allowing for ex-directory subscribers, there are very few of us. Identity thieves prefer more common names, because other people are less likely to remember them when they use a stolen credit card in a shop."

"So do you think we'll all be much safer with the proposed identity card system?" asked Anita, herself a total sceptic.

"Not at all, we'll be much less safe," said Matthew. "Imagine criminals getting their hands on all that data held by the government. Just think what they could do with it."
"And government departments are notoriously lax in that respect;" said Anita. "Remember the disks and memory sticks that went missing, as well as the printed documents left in cars or on trains, not to mention those whose top-secret contents were picked up by the long-lens-paparazzi, only to compromise an MI5 sting."

"In any case," said Matthew, " I'm against the government controlling my identity in that way, in principle." Anita smiled,
"You know what ***Joe Public*** keeps saying, 'I'm quite happy to purchase an ID card if it makes sure the criminals get caught. Folk must have something to hide if they're against ID cards.' Don't they realise what they are giving up? Similarly, government departments collaborating for a change, does, on the surface, sound like a good idea. It saves you having to fill out forms several times over asking for the same information. But don't people see how easily such information could be misused? Personal medical histories shared with insurance companies who only want your premiums if you're very unlikely ever to claim; financial information as well as spending patterns monitored by government departments to identify those pariahs who ***refuse*** to get into debt."
"Yes," said Matthew, isn't ironic that when the country's bankrupt, all they want us to do is acquire more debt to keep the economy afloat? You can imagine the latest disincentive-to-saving policy, can't you? Let's charge the customers interest on their unspent money: the more they save, the harsher the penalty."

In order to retrieve his soul, Matthew needed courage. A battle lay ahead, and he needed to experience what it was like to be a warrior. As a child, he was to learn the rudimentary skills.

## Chapter six – the fighter

Preparation for the adult world began for Matthew around the age of six in the local park. Here he learned, contrary to what his parents and every other authority figure (such as teachers and clergy) had told him, that fighting was good. It was a way of establishing your ranking in the pecking order, and even if you came out bottom of the heap, it was still an incentive to learn the tricks of the trade. Boxing was not an option, because none of the kids could afford boxing-gloves, but wrestling became the fighting-style of choice, before some of the kids started going to jujitsu lessons, that is. It was not until his adult years, when the sceptic overtook the believer, that he realised much of the action by 'professionals' on TV had been faked. However, Mick McManus had been the kids' wrestling hero of the day.

"Are you paid?" came the familiar question, as Matthew was eventually pinned down in a hold from which there was no chance of recovery. Despite losing most of his fights, Matthew later found the training it gave him invaluable, and he never totally forgot that adrenaline rush that spurred him on to future victories, with his favourite move, the bear-hug. As he matured, he realised that winning a fight did not solve a problem, and, coming off most often the loser rather than the winner in such contests, he soon learned to develop alternative more effective weaponry in the form of humour and words.

An adrenaline rush used to be essential for survival in the wild, enabling us to stand and fight where necessary, but also permitting us the option to run away, where we deemed discretion the better part of valour. Unfortunately, in many twenty-first century encounters, neither of these two options is appropriate. Primitive man would have picked up excrement and hurled it at his enemy. Civilised man substituted invective for faeces and this continues to this day in the choice of scatological swear-words. Matthew rarely used swear-words, except inside his head, when internal conflict prompted one of his inner demons to torment and lambaste him with scathing comments about his ineptitude.

"Stupid idiot!" one of them would comment, fairly innocuously, when he accidentally came off his bike. Then the other demons would join in, chanting in carefully coordinated cacophonous chorus, "What an arsehole, gormless wanker, he's crap at everything he tries to do!" Matthew resisted these voices that had plagued him since childhood, addressing them with the confidence of one who believes them to be simply an echo of the taunts of bullies at school or hypercritical teachers. He had to deal with them because they threatened every new venture he took on. He sometimes felt it was just a self-destructive streak that he recalled from the times when, after hours of painstaking precision gluing, he had smashed the practically complete model aeroplane to pieces, in a fit of exasperation. Perhaps destructiveness was part of the necessary baggage that accompanied creativity, he reflected.

Matthew often wondered why it was that an altercation between two working-class blokes usually ended up with a spell inside for both of them, whereas a similar argument between middle-class geezers generally resulted in a fine, a caution, or in most cases, no punishment at all. He put it down to vocabulary (and money) in the end.
"Middle-class geezers just don't come over as villains, do they?" Matthew asked Andy, the detective. "Why do they always get away with it?" Andy cited the judicious use of solicitors as the probable reason,
"And the rich know how to impress the judge and feign contrition. The working-class blokes don't exactly try very hard to impress. They may wear a suit, but they look so uncomfortable in it, and their inability to communicate, as well as their perceived disdain for the court, has them convicted before they have a chance to defend their conduct."

Matthew liked to think that he had moved fairly seamlessly from working-class to middle-class, but his wife thought otherwise,
"You're still an interloper," said Anita. "You still ask for permission to enjoy what is yours as of right. With your university education, you've earned some of the perks that accompany the talents you have developed. But you can't get rid of it, can you? You still have that working-class chip on your shoulder." Coming from the union of a working-class father, Arthur, and a middle-class mother, Edna, Matthew felt he had always had a foot in both camps. His links to working class values were very tenuous, though he was a life-long defender of the underdog. From his mother's interest in literature and the arts he had aspired to be free of peers who would mock anything that smacked of intellectualism and who cared for little apart from football, beer and women, in that order, and at weekends usually a punch-up.

## Chapter seven – the soldier

War is ugly, it is true, but it seems that you only feel truly alive when you are right on the edge, close to death. It was once claimed that the people of Northern Ireland were – despite the troubles – the happiest group in the United Kingdom, with a lower than average suicide rate.

Matthew had often wondered what it would have been like to be in the forces. His father's eyes had always lit up whenever he described World War Two experiences in North Africa and Italy. It was not until he visited these countries for himself that Matthew was able to capture – however vicariously - some of the excitement his father had witnessed. There had inevitably been casualties amongst his family members after WW2, though these were more of a psychological nature. On both sides of the family, individuals suffered – as his mother put it – 'with their nerves'. Of course, at the time it was very much taboo to even mention the word ***insanity***.

He had once played a game called ***Strategy*** with some American top brass and was somewhat amused that of the five colours you could choose from, the General would always go for white, or occasionally, blue, associating the red, yellow and black with inferior beings. The object of the game was to build alliances with other blocks in order to gain world domination. An alliance might be purely strategic and temporary: the aim was to annihilate the opposition. Nowadays, the military themselves play all-too-realistic three-dimensional war games. One wonders if they have sufficient grip on reality to divorce this fantasy world from the theatre of war.

On another occasion, he had talked with Ken, a bomb disposal officer, and realised how, as a soldier, you have to think more like a terrorist in order to second guess his next move. Simple chemistry allowed everyday household products and garden requisites, such as weed-killer, to become explosives. Knowing the potential dangers inherent in not having lockable fuel-caps, for example, could avoid the possibility of someone producing a lethal cocktail by adding something as commonplace as sugar or fertiliser to the petrol tank. Of course, today you do not have to have a knowledge of basic chemistry to know these things: the internet offers anyone curious enough to search for them the exact recipes for making bombs. Ken's job was a curious mixture of talents that emphasised the interaction of creation and destruction. As an engineer, his job was to construct bridges; yet, he might equally be required at any given time to blow them up. (A rock musician might find a similar irony in taking the instrument he had carefully had custom-built being smashed to pieces in some vaguely cathartic frenzy).

In the late nineteen-sixties, just at the time when Matthew's cohort was going off to college, the students seemed to have become radicalised, like many of the Asian students today – only back then it was Tariq Ali who inspired us. Matthew had his own pet single issues in politics, though he had been on a variety of demonstrations. The Grosvenor Square march against the Vietnam War had felt a perfectly laudable cause at the time. Thank goodness Harold Wilson had made the sensible decision in refusing to get our troops involved, he thought.

Later decades produced students with hardly a political bone in their bodies, but nowadays, it is primarily the Muslim students who are getting radicalised. Matthew could, with hindsight, understand the attraction of radicalism for that age-group.

One night in Kassel, he had met up with a group of similarly radicalised German students. Now, to understand the dissatisfaction of this group, one needed to appreciate that the two main political parties in the German Federal Republic had formed a coalition for the previous thirteen years. Effectively, this meant that whoever you voted for, you got the same bunch as before, who all had a vested interest in preserving the status quo - a right-of-centre alliance. Wolfgang and Dieter were not quite as extreme as some of the Bader Meinhoff members, but they spoke eloquently about the aims of the red army faction (RAF) and extra-parliamentary opposition (APO).

Yes, it was exciting doing something subversive. Leading up to the escapade, the local kids had met up to concoct some smoke bombs and prepare for the forthcoming graffiti. Matthew went along for the ride. He sat in the car whilst Wolfgang and Dieter produced what was later to be referred to as either Malerei (artwork) by the students, or Schmiererei (daubings) by the authorities. He had not for one moment imagined that there would be severe repercussions.

He was summoned by the local CID (Kripo) and asked to translate the message that had been painted on the wall, where a big military (Bundeswehr) procession was to pass by the next day. The CID must have thought he had committed this crime!

***Take a trip, look around, see the pigs that run your town.***

It was not till he got the chance to see Wolfgang and Dieter again, that he discovered the lines came from a Frank Zappa (Mothers of Invention) song. Having made a stab at the translation, he was asked to name names, being threatened with the fact that he would face a charge of perjury if he failed to incriminate the culprits, with the consequence that he would acquire a criminal record and never be allowed to teach again. What could he do? He decided to betray his friends.

The lawyers from ***linke Hilfe*** subsequently found him an exit strategy: since no interpreter had been present at his cross-examination, the evidence was deemed inadmissible. Doris provided him with a bed for the night and the following day he absconded to Greece for six weeks, somewhere he could lie low. (We shall here more of Doris in due course).

---

It was not until later on in his life that he discovered how the armed forces had appropriated certain psychological techniques used for heightening the awareness of soldiers in the field. He accidentally stumbled on the purpose behind keeping soldiers awake for long periods of time during one of his manic phases. He remembered Sylvia mentioning his hypersensitivity on another occasion, but this time it was not simply some kind of intuition about past atrocities: it was a super-awareness of what was going on all around him. For once in his life he felt truly alive. Mundane reality, in comparison, was more like being in a coma. There was not only that high degree of 'arousal', as the psychologists call it, where he could hear distant traffic sounds and also pick up aromas from miniscule traces of fragrances around the house, with all the lingering memories these evoked. More than this, he found he could see symbolic meanings in paintings - an ability which he had not had, in any way, previously. Even more fascinating was the synaesthesia that allowed him to hear colours and feel flavours. (cf the language we use in everyday speech: 'that's a loud colour' or 'that's got a sharp taste.')

Matthew realised how crucial this super-awareness was to a soldier on the alert for the enemy approaching. On the other hand, he seriously questioned the rationality of the manic mind: if patients take dangerous risks when they are ***hyper,*** would that not suggest that soldiers might react with a similar lack of judgement? As Matthew was quick to discover, when patients hit the manic phase of their bipolar cycle, they are deemed incapable of rational thought, and forbidden from driving cars or accessing their financial resources.

But Matthew liked this energetic and dynamic side of his personality, and so he thought it was time to don a suitable mask and go under cover.

## Chapter eight – the spy

***No need to inform us - we already know:***
***Soon everyone will have a chip on their shoulder.***
***(JS / 2005)***

Sue was never quite sure whether Matthew was telling the truth,
"It's all sounding a bit like Walter Mitty," she said after another of their regular sessions, "Were you really a spook?" Matthew was non-committal,
"Studying languages provides a good basis for becoming a spy. In a sense, you are already able to develop your ***alter ego*** and to reinvent yourself as a totally different personality. Generally speaking, there are only a few individuals who are genuinely bilingual in the sense that they can adopt the stereotypical persona of a particular nationality as well as speak the language fluently. What often gives the novice spy away is, ironically, the very perfection of his speech. What you quickly realise is that to be a ***plausible*** individual, you need the right mixture of dialect, sociolect and idiolect."

"Once I had actually resided in a region of Germany for two years, I had learnt to incorporate some of the local dialect words, the mild expletives, the level of intellectuality expected of a man of my calibre, as well as some of the mannerisms that native Germans might display. In those days, at a time when non-ethnic Germans stuck out like a sore thumb, I was frequently mistaken for an Austrian – at least this demonstrated that my spoken German was reasonably convincing. With a full head of blond hair, a full beard and blue eyes, I looked about as Germanic as the next man. However, I did have to draw the line when it came to wearing Lederhose and a Tyrolean hat with a feather in it!

I experimented with impersonations. One evening, I caught the tail-end of an interview in German with a Scot, describing an encounter with the Loch Ness Monster:

***Ich wartete drei Minuten, bis das Ungeheuer aus dem See kam.***

I practised perfecting the exact mixture of High German overlaid with Scottish intonation. Judging by the reaction from my German friends, the impersonation was quite convincing."

Sue was still unsure whether this was the truth, so she decided to put him to the test, "Who were you working for?" Matthew gave an instantaneous response,
"The Stasi - East German State Security Police - were tipped off by a mole working within my University that I would make the ideal "sleeper", based on my communist sympathies and relative lack of any significant criminal

record with the authorities back in England. At that stage, I was merely informed that I would be contacted at some unspecified future date by a current acquaintance. It was something of a shock to me when out of the blue I received a phone-call some fifteen years later from my former tutor at London University. The latter had been informed that I would be visiting Berlin and suggested that I drop in on him when I made the planned day excursion to East Berlin. My tutor had always put – shall we say – a more left-wing slant on his analysis of the great classical German writers and had eventually decided to move to the German Democratic Republic, an environment where his ideas were more in tune with those of the communist leaders than those of the Thatcher regime that had started to dominate the lives and attitudes of people back in England. This was all happening in the mid-1980's – just prior to the fall of the Berlin Wall in 1989."

Matthew had always secretly fancied the idea of being a spy. Not particularly for ideological reasons. It was more the romantic notion associated with clandestine affairs and - to be honest – the adrenaline rush experienced every time he came close to being caught out. His first assignment was not a complicated one. Prior to 1989, Germany had functioned as two separate countries with diametrically opposed ideologies. There had been some attempts to develop a kind of détente purely for practical reasons, and visits by the then Heads of State to each other's countries occurred on a sporadic basis. The East German leader was due to visit Kassel, a town quite close to the border, and it was to be Matthew's task to attempt to breach local security so that – if he was successful in getting through the police checkpoints - the Communist regime could gain a propaganda coup in demonstrating how lax the security in the Federal Republic was.

Matthew did the obligatory reconnoitre of the terrain. ***Wilhelmshöhe*** was a challenging venue. He contacted his West German student friends who were generally disenchanted with their government. He had to be sure that they would not betray him like he had been forced to betray others, previously. The plan was simple. He would use all his manipulative talents to persuade them that the idea was theirs and that he was just going along with it to humour their sense of childish fun.

Hans was key to all this. He was the one student who exuded confidence. His father, a rich industrialist, had just bought him a new car. Volker and Connie completed the party. What was the easiest way to pass reasonably smoothly through the police checkpoints, they wondered? Then Hans had a brainwave: they would be a team of rookie journalists. Hans quickly acquired – he never told them where from – an official-looking ***Presse*** sign which he displayed on his windscreen.

But first of all, they had to attempt to breach security without the sign, just to see how hard it might be.
"Nice try!" said the policeman at the first checkpoint. He was very friendly, and in view of the freezing temperatures that day he actually shared some of his soup with them (***Bullensuppe*** as his fellow passengers called it). Sitting and watching various cars and buses pass through, they noted that those displaying the "press" sign were waved through without much fuss. It was time to try their luck.

Surprisingly enough, they sailed through without difficulty and parked up alongside the other journalists. Mission successful. However, in order to prove to his East German handlers that he had successfully breached security, he needed to make sure his face was shown as part of the entourage on German television. He stood right next to some BBC journalists and felt an almost compelling desire to divulge to them how he had come to be there, but he kept calm, remembered his assignment and waited for the East German leader to appear.

There he stood, barely one metre away from the man. Had he been working for the other side, he could have taken him out, no sweat. Still, now it was time to go back to the flat and watch the replay first on east, and then west TV. (Living so close to the border, both stations were accessible to him). First of all, he watched the East German footage. Yes, there he stood, right next to the visiting Head of State. His handlers would be pleased with a job well done. The commentary ran along the lines:

***Despite reassurances to the contrary, it is quite clear that the West German authorities were incapable of sustaining even the most basic security around our esteemed leader.***

Turning over to the other transmitter, Matthew heard the anticipated denials of incompetency, and insistence that the local police and other security forces had acquitted themselves admirably.

Matthew could see how a person like himself, with no particularly strong views in favour of either side, might become a double-agent. However, he thought better of it and elected to play the part of messenger, instead.

## Chapter nine – the diplomat

Matthew had always found it difficult to take sides. Though he felt he knew instinctively what was right and what was wrong, he always listened to both sides of an argument and could rarely make up his mind which side to take. This character trait carried over to everyday life to such an extent that he often felt paralysed into inaction: the pros and cons as well as the consequences occupied his thoughts so completely. This, of course, tended to make him indecisive. It even extended to his voting intentions – quite often he would turn up at the voting station resolved to support one party only to change his mind at the last minute, casting his vote for a party at the opposite extreme.

As a child, he had tried to tread a careful path, trying hard not to annoy either party in a dispute. To some extent he succeeded, much as the potential victim of bullies develops a sense of humour to gain acceptance. But as an adult, this behaviour, he discovered to his cost, was frowned upon. His wife had wanted someone to protect her, ***whether she was right or wrong***, as the Bob Dylan song puts it; but again and again, he had tried to see the other person's point of view instead of demonstrating loyalty to her.

Matthew reflected on his behaviour: had it been simply cowardice, a desire to avoid confrontation at all costs? He liked to think not. After all, it often cost him dearly not to go with the flow: he felt that his motivation was always to hear both sides of an argument and to challenge what he thought was wrong. He frequently found himself on the side of the underdog, fighting for some universally recognised lost cause, going against the flow. How much easier it would have been to acquiesce, indeed to voice the odd word of support for the predominant view: it might not have alienated so many potential allies.

When he was working at a college in Glasgow in 1998, his boss, Bert, once had a heart-to-heart with him, elucidating the painfully uncomfortable change from union activist to middle management worker,
"I had once experienced the same difficulties in adjusting to my new role in management. Fraternising with the troops was no longer an option: it undermines corporate solidarity." However, Bert's recommendation to avoid socialising with his colleagues was a step too far for Matthew: he favoured a structure that promoted one community – not an ***us-and-them*** culture. He always believed that unity is strength and that isolated individuals are more easily picked off.

Bert continued,

"You people in middle management are like footballs: you get kicked from both sides - top-down and bottom-up. Of course, middle managers can pull rank and get support from senior management, provided they themselves tow the party line. The "kick-the-dog" syndrome can work." Matthew recalled being trained for such practices whilst still at school,
"Masters would delegate prefects to inflict unconventional punishments on younger pupils," he said. "The latter, in turn, were expected to console themselves with the certainty that when they themselves were promoted to the status of prefects, they would be able to exact revenge on the next unsuspecting cohort of boys."

There had been a logical hierarchy within this - at the time - unfathomable system of appointing prefects. Thugs were generally exalted to the status of Head Prefect and given virtually ***carte blanche*** to mete out whatever punishment they deemed appropriate and this, of course, included corporal punishment in those days. Matthew, because he did not show any potential on the sadistic scale himself, never made it any higher that toilet monitor, a role not exactly coveted by any of the non-prefects.

Bert remarked latterly that the role of ***diplomat*** suited Matthew quite well,
"Being blessed - or cursed - with a love of language and a way with words, you have learned how to re-interpret instructions, putting them into a form perhaps more palatable with the troops. Simply repeating word-for-word the instructions of your superiors fails to achieve the desired effect, probably because this is not in tune with your personality.

Some managers are expected to bark instructions like a dog: others have to adopt traits more commonly associated with the fox. It takes a degree of persuasion – some might say manipulation – to get folk to sing from the corporate hymn sheet. A manager can put on a variety of disguises. Yes, you can attempt to rule through fear, but ultimately, this needs to be replaced with mutual respect, otherwise even the tyrant will eventually become a laughing-stock. You can take the altruistic route and lead by example. You can call in return favours, if you want to be that cynical, but you have to be sincere in what you do, or you will quickly be found out. Your colleagues understand, of course, that the way you put across an argument to management will differ in presentation, certainly, if not in substance from the manner you deliver it to the team, but they will rightly resent you if you are totally two-faced."

Bert continued,
"To be a good diplomat you need to avoid foot-and-mouth disease: so when you open your mouth, don't put your foot in it. There is another danger, however, namely that you get so used to finding euphemisms and roundabout ways of hinting at the intended message, that those you are addressing - quite understandably - fail to receive it. The introductory and

concluding remarks stick, whilst the 'meat' in the shit sandwich (which was the negatively critical message you were intending to convey) is gulped down without any perceivable acknowledgement of its significance."
"I think I see," said Matthew.

"Then why don't you use plain English?" asked Bert, "Are you just trying to impress the audience with long words, or is it just part of your condition?" Matthew acknowledged that he often preferred flowery language, and that communication was often inhibited by the injudicious use of polysyllabic synonyms,
"I'll try harder in future," he said. "It does appear to be a common symptom of the illness. It goes along with an aloofness and a perceived unwillingness to participate socially, apparently."

Matthew did nevertheless learn how to hone his skills in this area. He liked being the man-in-the-middle. He could play devil's advocate, mediator or medium, the interpreter, the translator, the reporter and the peacemaker equally well. Naturally, in these roles he was frequently singled out as the target of abuse, sometimes verbal, but occasionally physical abuse. He knew that harbingers of truth had the habit of being shot at. However, it had often been his diplomacy (i.e. knowing when to keep ***stumm*** and listen for a change) that had successfully de-escalated many an argument that looked like turning nasty.

## Chapter ten – the interpreter

Many of the subtle nuances of the original texts often get lost in translation, which is, however, not true in the case of Hitler's ***Mein Kampf***, which some say was actually enhanced when it came to be translated. Matthew was particularly conscious of his innate desire to elaborate, exaggerate and embroider the original text, whenever faced with either a translation, or more frequently in recent years, a summary of a text. This made him acutely aware that no word really has an exact synonym, and even if it had, you could not prevent the reader from bringing along to the process their own connotations, acquired perhaps from painful ***associations*** with any given word.

Judging by its Latin roots, an ***interpreter*** seems to have acted as an intermediary between two merchants wishing to bargain around an agreed price, or ***pretium***. Foreign language skills may have been an added advantage whenever trading occurred between people from opposite ends of the Earth who did not share a common language. As we may recall, this kind of role appealed to Matthew. He enjoyed decoding as much as he enjoyed encryption, as he could fulfil the role of intermediary in an exemplary fashion.

One day, ***La belle Hélène*** came to him in desperation, when all she'd got back from the helpline was 'RTFM'! It transpired that the manual in question was constructed in a manner that defied logic. Only after reading its entire contents did the poor reader discover that the novice needed to start reading mid-way through the book. The earlier stuff assumed an advanced level of technological understanding that only technological experts would have understood, and, as we all know, they wouldn't have demeaned themselves so low as to actually read any such manual!

"I quite often find myself asked to decipher instruction manuals," said Matthew.
"You make it all sound so simple," said Helen.
"Well, it should be, really. It's just that the folk that put instruction manuals together don't understand the basic facts about communicating. If they were only to ask themselves who the potential audience was for the manual and what the purpose of providing the manual was in the first place, it would be a start, I suppose. Better still, they could employ the services of an interpreter to help demystify their jargon. Half the time, they're just trying to dress it up in fancy terminology anyway, so that we'll think they're smart and hence offer them due respect."

"Is it the same with all this academic twaddle I'm expected to regurgitate?" asked Helen.

"Let's have a look," said Matthew. Helen handed him an article by an eminent professor.
"***Individual Entropy***, now there's a concept ripe for deconstruction," said Matthew, "I take it you've looked at all the secondary literature, as well as comments on the internet?"
"Yes, I've done all my homework, but I just can't get my head round it," said Helen. "Sometimes it helps to compare your take on it with someone else's," said Matthew, "that way, you can judge whether your interpretation chimes in with theirs. If it does, you'll go away more certain in your understanding; whereas if it doesn't, at least you'll realise where you part company from them and you'll be able to look at it again from their point of view."

## Chapter eleven – the intermediary

With hindsight, Matthew realised his talents lay in communication and, with one foot in this world, and the other 'elsewhere', he felt he could deliver important messages to humanity. He was drawn to the roles of both medium and media, which both, in their own individual ways, bridged the gap between reality and fantasy / imagination.

The church had originally decided, in its infinite wisdom, to appoint individuals who could act as a bridge between life on Earth and the more celestial realms. The Pope was called in Latin ***pontifex maximus***, meaning a person who can provide a bridge between Heaven and Earth. Now, although Matthew had, as a child, exhibited something of an angelic disposition, he could never have claimed to be a saint, certainly not since he hit his late teens. Nevertheless, he did secretly feel somehow special, the anointed one. He realised quite early on that he seemed to possess some degree of intuitive ability more commonly associated with the female of the species.

Toying with graphology, Matthew initially thought it could all be put down to some scientific analysis of pen-strokes, and he set about mapping character traits against handwriting styles. It did appear that varying slant, spacing, zones, pressure, etc., did give an indication of the writer's personality, but ultimately, he found this clinical analysis unsatisfactory. Instead, he decided to put his own theory to the test. He believed that writers communicate with readers not only through their choice of words, but also through their script.

Ricky, a somewhat cynical colleague, agreed to hand him the middle pages of a hand-written letter. This excerpt would take away obvious clues such as the identity and gender of the writer. Matthew abandoned the scientific analysis and cleared his mind, as far as he could, of any preconceptions about the subject. Subconsciously, he asked the writer to reveal himself / herself, as he read and re-read the two pages. Now, any charlatan can exploit gullible punters by telling them what they want to hear. You only need to select generalisations and flattering comments. What makes a reading all the more credible is a situation where some home truths are being delivered. "Rubbish!" exclaims the subject in response to some derogatory comment. "But that ***is*** you!" respond his (or her) colleagues, practically in unison.

Anyway, back to the reading. The writer was definitely a female. What came across – and this was not in any way revealed in the actual words of the letter – was a deeply troubled individual with schizophrenic tendencies. Matthew's colleague was amazed. Ricky had deliberately chosen this person's handwriting for analysis as he had assumed she would present more of a conundrum. Instead, Matthew had identified the lady without difficulty. Ricky, normally the sceptical scientist, was somewhat disconcerted.

It was often difficult functioning as an intermediary, particularly when you were operating between two universes. With – metaphorically – one foot in this world and the other foot in a totally different domain, inhabited (if that was the right word) by shadowy characters with hidden agendas, Matthew sometimes found it impossible to concentrate sufficiently and was awakened from his reverie by some initially distant voice asking if he was paying attention or having what is rather disparagingly referred to as a 'senior moment'.

After taking a passing interest in film, Matthew got to play two characters on the screen. On the first occasion, he was, he felt, type-cast as a medieval priest whose task it would be to exorcise a demon:

***"In the name of the Almighty, get ye gone, ye spirits of evil."***

The short amateur production, filmed in Bury in the nineteen-eighties, and now immortalised on DVD, took three years to complete and included a short scene where his daughter Kate had played the witch's associate, carrying her little book of spells.

Matthew was subsequently identified by a production company for Channel Four to play the role of tree scientist. Although he would appear in the programme for less than thirty seconds, he took the opportunity very seriously, and even went to the ridiculous extent of trying out method acting.
"If I am to be convincing in this part, I need to look and act the part", he told his wife, Anita.
"All right, she reluctantly replied, "Let's get you the appropriate outfit."

Next he needed to do the recce and identify the props.
"Now, bear in mind that this drill you'll be holding is a very expensive piece of kit", explained Eric, the Danish director.
"How much is it worth?" asked Matthew.
"Around £20,000," replied the director. From that point onwards, Matthew resolved to research the device in great detail. Apparently, this drill enabled its operator to assess the age and condition of the wood, regardless of the age of the tree. The drill was connected to a device that gave the equivalent of an ECG for human beings. Looking at the read-outs, he could see that harder layers offered greater resistance, and this was reflected in the squiggles on the read-out. Softer layers were more quickly penetrated and

hence displayed different squiggles. To find a suitable oak tree for the scene the film crew had ventured into the depths of Sherwood Forest.

Matthew had not realised the extent to which strict demarcation lines existed between actors and technicians, until he offered to help one of the crew with his Paganinis.[9] The only time when everyone came together on an equal footing was the point where sandwiches emerged. Two days filming for less than thirty seconds on screen: what a lot of waste was involved. With video, he would probably have re-used many of the tapes, but each eleven minute reel of film seemed like a tremendous extravagance. The director explained that he was looking for quality images, and that these could only be produced using film, not video.

It was not until the film had its premiere in Manchester that Matthew got to meet the other actors. Each scene had been shot at a time and place to suit the participants' heavy schedules. Getting famous soap stars to front the programme had been quite a coup. But it was Mavis, the medium, who particularly interested Matthew. He had seen her perform her tree-hugging ritual and contemplated its significance. Perhaps this was yet another "bridge" that human beings could tap into, this time a means of communicating not with another place, but with another time. Just imagine what changes those thousand-year-old trees in America would have witnessed. How well they had learnt to adapt to environmental and climate change. Matthew leaned back against the gigantic great oak that had been chosen for his scene in the film 'Reunion'. Mavis had explained the thinking behind tree-hugging, and he tried to conjure up all the memories his tree retained.

He knew that human memories existed not solely in the brain, but more commonly in our muscles, bones and sinews. Playing the same tune over and over again with the jazz band had taught him that. He had heard of people receiving transplants allegedly inheriting the characteristics of their donors, too. The same thing seemed to work with old buildings that retained in the silicon compounds of their stone structures recordings of past traumatic events which they replayed from time to time, just to scare the new occupants. Since the tree was a living thing, how much more likely was it that past events had been recorded within its very soul? After all, the rings gave an indication of its age. (Like the ice-cores obtained from the Arctic that could show our history going back to Roman times, and with clear indications from the deposits within the ice of the time the industrial

---

[9] Blocks of wood carried on poles that are used to make outdoor settings level for filming purposes. They are placed underneath the track that the camera travels along.

revolution began.) This thousand-year-old specimen had survived plague and pestilence, war and famine.

"Trees will give us the first signs that our planet is dying," warned Mavis, "Like our own liver, they can handle a remarkable level of toxicity – and that's why we get so many effective remedies for our illnesses from trees – but even trees reach a point where they can't survive, whether it's due to acid rain, drought, pollution, or any number of other causes that mankind is ultimately responsible for through his thoughtless stewardship of the Earth."

For obvious reasons, an alpha male does not want to entertain any notion that he might only be a ***medium***. However, Matthew was quite surprised to hear that male mediums did exist. In his experience, it had tended to be females who performed this role, and there seemed to be a variety of motivations behind their selection of this profession. One had shown a remarkable gift for identifying locations for future jobs for Matthew. She had, equally impressively, accurately named individuals, like Kenny and David, who were to feature quite prominently in his future life, ten years later. Had this become a self-fulfilling prophesy, the cynic within him wondered? He didn't believe so. Yet another palm-reader had rightly predicted his change of direction towards more creative pursuits. Mavis, on the other hand, had been ***spot on*** when it came to communicating with those who had recently deceased. Matthew's mother, who had passed away only a matter of months before his sitting with Mavis, was quite clearly identifiable - as his wife agreed - right down to her slippers, mannerisms and foibles. Mavis suggested that Matthew's daughter had what Mavis called "the gift". Matthew wondered if Kate would ever put it to use.

Kate was an enigma, in many ways. Matthew always liked to remember her from her days in primary school, having had little sustained contact with her in recent years, living as he did some five hundred miles away from her home. She was a really attractive young woman, as he could see from the odd photograph he had received from her mother. Like himself, she was equally capable of being very kind or very cruel, and again, parallel to his own veritable army of characters, she inhabited several personae at different times.

## Chapter twelve – the editor

Matthew continued to pursue his interest in film. This fantasy world very much appealed to him. He would sit, often for hours on end, carefully matching up the video clips in his edit suite, blissfully unaware of the passage of time. He was now living in the Highlands of Scotland, playing with his new expensive toy. He marvelled at the way longer edits would artificially slow down time, whilst clips with a duration of less than a second, once spliced together in a sequence, would speed it up. (Witness the use of the former in love scenes and the latter in action movies.)

As he sped the tape forwards and backwards to find the crucial editing point, Matthew wondered what effect the whole process was having on his eyes, and tangentially on his brain. No health and safety time limits were placed on the video editing sessions: he devoted as much or as little time to the tasks in hand as he chose, because he enjoyed them. He likened the experience to the early days of motor vehicles, where it was assumed that the speed at which you could safely drive must be determined by the rate at which the brain could process incoming data in the form of random images. We all now know that much of our driving is carried out effectively on automatic pilot, and when asked to recall our journey, only certain memorable events come to mind.

Driving the desk was similar. Matthew could process the gist of what was taking place at fifteen or more times the twenty-five frames a second filming speed. Of course, he could not catch the soundtrack even if he slowed it down to fifty frames a second, when he heard what sounded like those old 'Alvin and the chipmunks' records. Matthew did once experience a strange consequence after sitting there too long: he continued to see after-images for some time after leaving the edit suite. They hung around in his peripheral vision.

He recalled the subliminal advertisements for Coca-Cola that were ultimately banned from the cinemas. It had been discovered that inserting one image of the beverage every so many frames actually increased sales of the drink during the interval. Unwitting punters had no idea they had been bombarded with this – admittedly - very effective form of advertising. Even today, messages flashing black on a white background then white on a black background can have a similar effect, though these seem to have slipped in under the radar of the Advertising Standards Authority.

With editing, he became something of control-freak. Having perused the delivery of speeches over and over again, he got to know all the performers, probably better than they knew themselves. He picked up on their every character trait. He could detect the care they had taken in rehearsing their lines. He could perceive all the rhetorical devices used, the deliberate pauses to allow for expected applause and the calculated exploitation of silence. The players became his marionettes, primed to dance to his tune.

Matthew had made a fleeting encounter with Prince Charles, when his media students filmed one of his annual visits to Scotland. Matthew had selected two students to do the filming, one male, and one female. When the security checks on the two were being conducted, he secretly anticipated that one might be rejected due to his noticeable Northern Ireland accent, since at the time, the troubles were at their height, and the security services must have imagined terrorists turning up in any manner of guises. However, the filming went to plan and the two students were delighted to get the chance to speak to the visitor. Matthew was impressed that HRH addressed every student by name during the interviews, clearly having done his homework prior to the visit.

Matthew's challenge was to get the video footage edited down and a DVD produced all in one day. This made him somewhat nostalgic for the past when the media did not have to be quite so im***media***te. The team's biggest headache was the usual editor's nightmare: the weather. Nobody wanted it to be a particularly sunny day – that itself can cause problems. Likewise, it would have been hard to brighten up the images if it had been a rainy day. The challenge was to edit together clips of video lasting seconds from footage filmed over a matter of hours in a climate where you can get four seasons in one day. Matthew particularly liked, from a technical point of view, the way the Prince's arrival outside the entrance to the college ***segued*** effortlessly into his appearance inside the foyer, despite the shower of hail.

Matthew was born in the same year as Charles, so he could relate back to comparable experiences at various points in their lives. He vividly recalled that they were both caught drinking underage: it was a rite of passage, a necessary rebellion, he felt. Only in Charles' case, the poison of choice had been cherry brandy when he was at Gordonstown , whilst Matthew's experience was in the rather less salubrious surroundings of a 'men only' pub in Dewsbury.
"Hard to imagine, in our PC world, isn't it?" said Matthew to his son, on the latter's annual visit north.

Mark had developed into a veritable pillar of society. About to experience fatherhood, Mark showed himself well able to provide for and look after his family. The resemblance between Mark and Matthew was uncanny: even down to their shared sense of humour. Mark's control-freakery, however, extended only to computers. As a computer manager, he was inherently suspicious of the operators, and preferred to restrict their access to many of the possible features, for fear that they might either bugger something up, or, alternatively, start working on their own projects in company time. His saving grace was that he refused to take this attitude home with him. The cheeky grin he met you with was contagious, and you found yourself inadvertently mimicking his smile.

"What was the experience like?" enquired Mark.
"As I recall, the experience was less than enthralling. Me and my mate, Gary, asked for two pints of Tetley's in our deepest bass voices. We had deliberately not shaved for the past week, but the bum-fluff on our upper lips could hardly have been convincing.
"There's a copper just walked in!" warned the barman.
"So what?" replied Gary, suddenly finding courage, though not of the alcoholic variety. The challenge had only been a bluff on the part of the barman and he, however reluctantly, pulled them the pints.

"Didn't they ask for your ID cards?" asked Mark, Matthew's son.
"They didn't exist in my day – actually, that's a lie – I found an ID in the loft that was issued to people immediately after the Second World War. Anyway, to paint you a picture of the interior of the pub, I need to get you to imagine what décor looks like when it has never had the benefit of a woman's touch. Everyone smoked then and the nicotine built up on the ceiling. The Clean Air Act hadn't yet come in, so some pretty sulphurous coal had added to the yellowing of the wallpaper. God knows what colour it was originally. The lower half of the wall was covered in ***Lincrusta*** that had been covered up at some point with some thick treacly-black varnish. Malodorous liquids of various hues and consistencies dripped slowly down the walls, and you could have been forgiven for wondering if you hadn't walked accidentally into a public urinal rather than a pub."

Prior to his breakdown, Matthew used to enjoy reading, or listening to the odd play on Radio Four. The absence of accompanying images served a worthy purpose: it enabled Matthew to use his imagination. Visualisation is an innate ability within all of us which the British began to use most effectively in their learning process until the Puritans came along and outlawed the practice, because they associated it with the devil's work. Nowadays it is back with a vengeance – no self-respecting educationalist would feel they were addressing the needs of those students with visual learning preferences without the obligatory PowerPoint Presentation.

Right back when it all began, when the Lumière brothers presented their film of a train coming into the station (to the consternation of the audience who dived for cover behind the seats), Hugo von Hofmannsthal had warned in his essay, ***Ersatz für die Träume***,[10] of the potential damage that film might cause to the psyche. Little could he have anticipated that human

---

[10] Substitute for dreams

beings only a century on would be acting out their second lives in cyberspace.

"You teachers need to experience life in the real world," one high-flying whizz-kid from the City had remarked. Matthew pondered the statement for a while. Here was this guy who spent all his time in front of a screen, speculating with futures and derivatives, asking Matthew to step into some surreal alternative world and abandon normal face-to-face interaction with his fellow human beings!

Film itself was a kind of twilight world. It seemed to Matthew that it was a way of substantiating ghosts, of rendering ordinary mortals immortal. Where we had previously relied on artists to hand down images of celebrities of yesterday, now we could relive their lives an infinite number of times, simply by playing back a video or DVD. It was as if we had succeeded in recording our mirror images for posterity. Suspending our disbelief even one stage further, we can now create and interact with extremely realistic-looking three dimensional avatars. Surely we are beginning to lose our grip on reality? Matthew himself was to experience a similar twilight world when he embarked on the rollercoaster ride that was his breakdown. Like many who stray into this fantasy existence, he soon began to doubt his sanity, finding it impossible eventually to differentiate between reality and non-reality.

Perhaps it was time to give images a rest, and concentrate, for a change, on sounds. But what kind of sounds? Leading up to his breakdown, the ***radio*** was his constant companion, specifically a twenty-four hour diet of Radio Four. After his breakdown, he experienced a subtle change in his listening habits: from now on it was Radio Two that predominated, mainly because he wanted music, not talk in his life. And yet, he had needed those background voices emanating from God knows where to help him get off to sleep. Without a woman to share his bed, he felt the need at least of communication in the form of sound, and the BBC World Service was to fulfil this need. However, Matthew kept going back to the words of the Helen Reddy song, Angie Baby. The notion of boy 'with evil on his mind' setting out to take advantage of the crazy girl, only to discover that she is actually more powerful than him was intriguing. In dreams, radio represents spiritual communication, and here it acquires almost a succubus attribute as the boy is sucked into the radio, only to be revived whenever Angie decides she needs his services. Radio must have seemed a truly spooky medium when it first appeared, with all its disembodied voices coming out of the ether. But just imagine the impact of being able to trap these voices on magnetic tape!

## Chapter thirteen – the recorder

Matthew kept no diaries: he relied almost exclusively on his photographic memory. He had a similar aversion to alarm clocks and had trained himself to awaken at exactly the right time every morning.
"Folk are far too dependent on unnecessary devices", he would say, "They should learn to be far more self-reliant". He had taken very few photographs over the years to plot the passage of his life. He already possessed an old movie projector which had to be cranked by hand. Turning the handle at a regular speed to get the picture sequence to run smoothly was an art in itself. However, his father had later bought him, in his teenage years, a matching second-hand movie camera which operated by clockwork. The film used was 9.5 mm. He had taken the camera with him to the Austrian Tyrol. The camera held out for the holiday, but on his return home the mainspring snapped. Still, he had succeeded in getting some footage for posterity. There were several classic silent films up in his loft – one of an early Disney movie with Mickey Mouse as Steamboat Willie. The cans of film lay side-by-side (as seemed appropriate) with a collection of old 78 rpm phonograph records.

Alongside the records were some reel-to-reel tapes on which he had once attempted to record his early songs. His Grundig machine produced its most faithful sound at seven-and-a-half inches per second. Already uncertain about entering into the teaching profession, Matthew felt he would have one last attempt at becoming a song-writer. He hawked his tapes up and down Denmark Street: London's Tin-Pan-Alley. All the recordings consisted of was his voice with guitar accompaniment. Perhaps he should have been more persistent, because apart from one outright rejection, most promoters did him the service of actually listening to the songs. If anything, the songs were deemed too original, and hence not commercial enough. One fellow actually wanted him to go away and write a song for Cliff Richard. Another suggested he copy the style of ***Storm in a Teacup***, one of the hit songs of the day, by the Fortunes.

Of course, once he had prostituted himself in that way, generating some catchy bubble gum sound, it was still not enough for them to make a final judgement.
"Go and get it recorded properly with session musicians, and then we shall see!" Needless to say, as a penniless student with no musical contacts to call on for any such favours, Matthew had reluctantly to abandon the idea. Years later, he felt inspired to give the next generation a chance of fame and took them down to ***Graveyard Sounds***, a recording studio in Manchester. At a reunion party, Matthew was delighted to meet one of the lads, Darren, who had eventually made it big-time working with Mike Oldfield and Gary Numan, as it transpired.

As will later be seen when we consider the multiplicity of roles he took upon himself, Matthew was in danger of becoming a jack of all trades – master of none. Indeed, he once got some good advice from Burkhart, a German businessman in the aviation industry.
"You'll never get promotion whilst you continue to try and augment your income in this way! – Look at you: you can hardly keep your eyes open. Do you have to work all the hours God sends?" Matthew had to admit that during that particular week, in additional to his full-time teaching commitment, he had put in twenty hours, labouring for his friend, Pete, a local builder. Not content with that, he had played in a band on two separate evenings. (One has to remark here that the band was clearly doomed to failure since the lead singer did shift work at the Mars chocolate factory in Slough. He came from Malta - no ***malteser*** jokes, please! - and was always asking the other members of the band if it was day ten yet: Mario worked three early shifts, followed by three late shifts and three night shifts ; days ten, eleven and twelve were his equivalent of what we would call a weekend. Unsurprisingly, agreeing on dates for gigs was a nightmare).

There came a time when Matthew was required, as part of his studies, to keep a reflective journal and we shall see later how this fortuitous memoire tracked his descent into madness as well as the first indications we have of his road to recovery. Apart from his letters that recipients had kept, there do not appear to be any other written records retained by Matthew.

Matthew was torn. One side of him was quite happy to retain the memories in his head; the other side of him wanted to commit pen to paper and record the events. It paralleled his desire to hoard material goods, whilst being a fervent believer in recycling. But then, life itself is a paradox, is it not?

## Chapter fourteen – the collector

Matthew had always been a hoarder. He just could not bear to throw anything away. He knew that people who had lived through hard times during World War Two were inclined to hoard things. Clearing away his mother's possessions after her death in 1994 at a hospital in Halifax, was an inherently sad experience, as he thought of all the treasured associations she would have had with so many of these inanimate objects – letters, postcards, ration books etc – he had to smile when he came upon several tins of ***carnation*** milk with a price tag of one-shilling-and-sixpence on them (sell-by / use by dates are a relatively recent requirement that those having to survive in more desperate times would have found an extremely wasteful idea). He also smiled on discovering some unopened Christmas presents: inside the wrapping paper was a pristine linen tea-towel, depicting a calendar for 1962. "Waste not, want not," he declared, echoing the motto he remembered his parents recite, and the towel is still in use at his home to the present day.

"Nobody collects things nowadays", he said to Anita, his wife, starting to feel angry about our throw-away culture.
"Looking through my mother's letters, I have to admit I felt a bit like a voyeur being offered such an insight into aspects of her life that had remained private and none of my business till today".
"You must keep the letters," said Anita. "They might well be fascinating for posterity." His mother, as he noted from her birth certificate, was born in 1905 and would have been forty-three when he was born in 1948. There were, of course, several children born immediately after the war for obvious reasons, many of them to older women, but the dangers of having children at this time of life may not have been so well understood then. It cannot have been an easy birth, needing as it did a forceps delivery.

"What shall I do with all her clutter?" he asked Anita, looking at clothes that had been the height of fashion in the nineteen-forties.
"You should donate most of them to local charity shops – and get the guy who runs the second-hand shop to take the remaining items of furniture from her flat."
"I suppose it's better these things get re-used", Matthew would say, "even if they end up in the hands of some rich antiques-collector." Matthew suddenly had what he thought was a profound thought.
"All the collections owned by wealthy families result from – shall we euphemistically say – acquisitions, often purloined from poorer people all over the world by intrepid adventurers: occasionally, for reasons generally other than philanthropic, the collections end up in the hands of the National Trust or municipal museums."

"So are you saying," Anita reflected, "that working class people don't hand down possessions from one generation to the next?"
"A few little trinkets, perhaps," said Matthew, "but most of what the surviving family members see as clutter disappears without trace, probably ending up eventually in the hands of some rich collector, or, worse still, as landfill."

He tried to imagine his own son and daughter sifting through his rubbish after his death,
"Do you think they will cherish the family heirlooms - such as war medals - as I did?" Anita was not so sure,
"Maybe putting the medals on E-bay will be one of the few remaining ways of converting possessions into cash now that the world economy is going into melt-down, saddling future generations with crippling debt. Whatever will they make of the bizarre contents of our loft?"
"Perhaps I need to provide a guide to the disposal of my assets," said Matthew, "At least they won't have the letters to sort through: nobody writes them nowadays." "How sad", said Anita, "E-mails leave no trace; we delete them. What evidence will remain - when we are gone - of our very existence? You must start writing a book."

"All these records we keep of our lives," said Matthew, "How will they be accessible to future generations? No good relying on obsolete technologies. Even within my lifetime, sound has gone from reel-to-reel recordings, through audio cassettes to CD's and now even they will become obsolete with little certainty of anyone being able to play the recordings back in a couple of generations' time. Hopefully there will be someone out there busying himself / herself with the archiving of sound materials for access by future historians. Again, it will only be the recordings of important people that will be kept; the lifetime contributions of the man-in-the-street will most probably be erased for ever, unless the archivist deems them admissible perhaps as a token ***vox pop*** element. I must have a word with Veronica, the archivist."

"What about all the video-recordings you have so painstakingly assembled?" said Anita, who, like Matthew, did not like wastage and had suggested they re-use the tapes in the spirit of recycling. Matthew had other ideas and retained over ten years' accumulation of footage. Of course, by this time, video was a redundant medium. "More useless clutter destined for the skip," said Anita.
"***Au contraire***. Another great bequest for posterity", said Matthew, assigning them to a convenient corner of his loft.
"They are going to have to be folk with an awful lot of time on their hands", said Anita, "Let's hope ***posterity*** has a multitude of little helpers, or they'll be cursing you for seriously wasting their precious time!"

"My mother's photographs!" said Matthew. "Now there's a lovely collection to inherit". His cousin, Liz, had always been a fount of information about all these Victorian-looking types that peered back at us from the albums. She could identify even the distant cousins, twice removed, as well as other categories of relative you never realised existed. Anita had to admit that photographs were a delight. She herself had a very good eye for taking a picture and had accumulated well into the thousands of images using her digital camera. She preferred to capture places as opposed to people, but Matthew always persuaded her to get one or two that included family members, just for posterity.
"What makes you think posterity will be remotely interested in my photographs", she mused.
"Well, put it this way", he replied, "most of us are fascinated by old photographs, and we seem to have an inbuilt desire to connect with our forebears in some way."

His memory had stood him in good stead, but Matthew needed to provide a tangible record of these so ephemeral experiences, whether a visual or a written record, it did not much matter.

## Chapter fifteen – the technician

Matthew got the uncontrollable urge to keep things, rather than throw them away; to repair things rather than replace them. Being a natural born fixer, Matthew took to the role of technician like a duck to water.
"How are we going to get our experiment to work out here in Holland?" enquired Alice. "It's only ever been tried out in the UK."

Alice and Matthew had been parcelled off on this jaunt to Holland just after Christmas in 1995. They had both recently been promoted, but had scarcely ever even met before the trip. She was quite tall, of athletic build and in possession of that same charisma that Matthew was later to observe whenever he approached the zenith of his mania. That is not to suggest that Alice was in any way unbalanced - far from it: Alice was to provide the very stability that Matthew so desperately needed. The relationship with one another remained platonic throughout their acquaintance.

"Leave it to me", replied Matthew, mischievously sensing that feeling of immunity all foreigners seem to experience abroad. The atmosphere had been extremely relaxed, especially after lunch when one of the delegates came back clearly stoned out of his mind. (This was Amsterdam, after all!). Matthew checked for sockets and quickly spotted that the telephone plugs in Holland looked more like British electrical plugs. The conference they had attended was supposed to be about sharing new technologies, but it soon became apparent to Matthew that here were issues beyond his sphere of influence. Once again he was to imagine the CIA at work, this time in industrial espionage. The French, according to his contacts in the information technology business, were making worrying advances in this field, and the Americans were in danger of lagging behind. Matthew knew it was going to be difficult getting the necessary plug. He had to find out, without making it too obvious what his reasons were, how to wire up the plug. Much as used to be the case with the GPO, the Dutch authorities did not like anyone other than their own telecoms employees tampering with the wires. There were four wires. Matthew felt a bit like a bomb disposal expert in his recently assumed Walter Mitty persona. "Trial-and-error!" he confidently proposed, getting Alice to collude in his subterfuge. First he unscrewed – thanks to the connivance of the Italian contingent - one of the plugs that was attached to their display. From this he could clearly see which wire connected to which prong. To cut a long story short, the experiment worked and communication was established, paving the way towards the international videoconferencing we all take for granted nowadays. (For obvious reasons, Matthew refrained from claiming the patent!).

Matthew's attitude towards computers was somewhat ambivalent: they were occasionally a useful tool, but frequently a huge waste of time. One activity did, however, simultaneously amuse and fascinate him and that was the ***defragmentation*** process. Spell-bound he watched, as the tiny coloured blocks were unceremoniously tossed into the air, only to come to rest in different configurations. By defragging his computer, he discovered, he could free up space.
"What an interesting idea!" mused Matthew, "I wonder if we could apply it to the brain? After all, many of the processes a computer goes through mirror those of our brains. Too much clutter - or at least disorganised strands of intermingled facts and feelings. Perhaps, like Aristotle, we need to categorise all this wealth of unrelated data. In that way, we can perhaps regain our sanity." Defragmentation was, indeed, the therapeutic process Matthew was ultimately to undergo with the help of his spirit-guide, Jean-Paul.

Matthew had never been even remotely inclined to tidy up. It was not sheer laziness that motivated, or rather de-motivated him in this enterprise. He needed to be able to ***see*** everything laid out in front of his eyes for any of it to be current in his working day. He had tried organising for himself a filing cabinet, but it had become redundant almost as soon as it had been set up, because he immediately forgot what was in it. A year later, he returned to check its contents and he could not remember why the various categories had been established at all. Matthew was no better at organising his files, now that they were to be kept electronically. Putting them all into folders effectively relegated them to oblivion, since he could not ***see*** their contents, and he had difficulty remembering what headings he had placed them under. All this interaction with machines was becoming very tedious. He devoted at least two days a week to the process and could not frankly see any benefit being derived from all that work.

"Out-of-sight, out-of-mind! I suppose", said Anita, reminding him of the contents of the loft. Momentarily adopting the persona of computer-translator, Matthew responded,
"Unsichtbarer Idiot![11]" convinced that a computer would never match the skills of a human translator, with our ability to spot nuances of meaning and idiomatic expressions.

However, once computers were finally accepted as an indispensible tool of the trade, Matthew decided to embrace them wholeheartedly. Never one to entrust the technical know-how to others, Matthew made a point of keeping up-to-date with all the latest advancements. He had mastered the intricacies of the professional edit suite, equipped with little more than the

---

[11] Allegedly the translation provided by a computer translation service (= invisible idiot)

manufacturer's handbook. It soon got round that if you wanted some technical problem fixing, Matthew was your man. Of course, in the early days, this did not exactly endear him to those whose job it was to fix such things, but later on, as technicians began to become increasingly remote from their fellow human beings, they were only too glad to have one thing less to fix, and even awarded him an 'honorary technician certificate' in recognition of his services.

Like most boys, Matthew had enjoyed taking things apart, but unlike the majority, he had particularly relished the challenge of putting them back together again. He had started with an old ***Napoleon*** clock that had belonged to his grandparents. First, he carefully removed the back. Then he started to brush away dust, dead flies and other debris that had accumulated over the years. Finally, he applied some three-in-one oil to the cogs and tentatively turned the key. At first there was no response. He gently touched the fly-wheel and it whirred into action. His first repair, a lovingly restored antique.
"Put a sock in it!" said his mother, after he had left the clock to perform the Westminster Chimes all night. It had gone off every quarter of an hour!

This fascination with the workings of everyday items had stood him in good stead when he was an impoverished young teacher with a young family to support. When the trusted ***Bendix*** washing machine finally surrendered to the onslaught of daily nappies, Matthew was in no mood to give in. There was no way they could afford to call in the repair man, let alone buy a new or reconditioned machine. He decided to methodically take it apart. After all, it was only a glorified motor, wasn't it? He removed sundry nuts and bolts to disengage the motor, reminding himself that he would have to ensure that the belt was at a suitable tension when he re-inserted the motor. The latter did not look to be in bad condition. When he removed the carbon bushes, he could see that they had worn right down. But where was he to purchase replacements?
"We only sell to trade!" asserted the man behind the counter, but then, realising from Matthew's face that this would not be an option, he suggested, sympathetically, "Might your business be ***A & A Repairs Ltd*****?"**

Matthew not only got his washing-machine running again: he went on to repair it for a further ten years by which time reconditioned motors had become more expensive than brand new washing machines. He relished the very challenge of replacing a timer with its fifty or so electrical connections. He remembered a trick he had learnt from a colour-blind would-be computer technician: each wire is usually printed with a specific identification number.

"Nobody likes a smart-arse!" commented Godfrey, a computer whizz-kid, after Matthew had found a simple solution to projecting video onto the recently installed cinema screens.
"It takes one to know one!" replied Matthew, dangling the short yellow-ended lead in front of Godfrey's eyes.
"Information is power", commented Godfrey.
"So, instead of your mushroom management – keep them in the dark and drop shit on them – how about sharing your information instead of being such a control-freak!" suggested Matthew.
"It takes one to know one", replied Godfrey.
"Touché!" acknowledged Matthew, left wondering why he enjoyed so much the experience of being needed - indispensible even.

## Chapter sixteen – the politician

"I'd always got you type-cast as a moderate," said Alan, who, as a life-long supporter of the Labour movement, was generally quite astute when it came to categorising people he encountered. "That's why I got you to play a ***moderate*** in Brecht's ***Days of the Commune***, but now I'm wondering if you might, in fact, be a crypto-fascist."
"Well, look at our society today. Have we really got it right about the way we bring up our kids? You probably think the abolition of corporal punishment was a good thing?" said Matthew.
"Don't tell me you want to go back to the bad old days where sadistic teachers got their daily kicks from caning their pupils?" said Alan.
"Well, you know what they always said, Alan, spare the rod[12] and spoil the child," said Matthew.

"It's all about back-scratching", observed Roy, one of the Conservative councillors, after a particularly lively debate. Matthew had represented the interests of his colleagues over a four year period in the early nineteen-eighties in Bury – probably well past the time when he should have automatically had to stand down. "Although both our legal system and our political system are adversarial, we do not necessarily have to set out with the objective of alienating the other side, despite what you may have observed today. You might think that the way to score Brownie points is to lay bare the hypocrisy of your opponent or to promote your own altruistic crusade for the underdog: that would be to seriously misjudge how committees, sub-committees and ad hoc working parties function."

"But I want to ensure that the truth comes out. I do not understand why everyone in politics seems to get corrupted. Is it all about money? Does every aspiring politician already have his or her pre-existing hidden agenda, or do they just get nobbled at some point in their ascendency by big business?"

"Every man has his price", remarked Councillor Williams, "Even you, despite your claim that no one could ever buy you off. It's not always about money. If you, for example, would prefer more recognition in your teaching role, I could arrange that for you, perhaps a promotion – not for the extra cash, though, of course, that might be a consideration, even for you. Find the Achilles Heel and you have already built up debt, only in this instance a debt of gratitude. Usually, maybe only at a subliminal level, the fish will have been hooked into owing you a favour. Eventually, the truth – whatever you may understand by that particular arbitrary concept – becomes the

[12] The term fascist originally comes from the Latin ***fasces*** meaning rods

casualty of expediency. Getting your voice heard isn't about gaining colleagues' respect for your sincerity and integrity: it's about the rather sickly sycophantic process of learning how to manipulate people by massaging their egos. You could start with the basics – you only have to indicate your agreement with any particular speaker through a comment such as 'I agree', but make sure your voice carries sufficiently to ensure that it is your individual endorsement he takes note of, not that of the crowd. Be seen to lead rather than follow the chorus of approval."

"So, why are you giving me all this advice, Councillor? After all, you are well aware that we are on opposite sides of the political divide."
"Nominally, perhaps that is true, but I have taken a close interest in the motivation behind your lines of thinking, and I believe that fundamentally we hold similar values".
"How could that be?" enquired Matthew.
"Imagine for a second – just suspend disbelief, if you like – imagine, as I say, that there really is just one objective reality or truth out there: how could we possibly all interpret it in the same way? One person will see it through rose-tinted spectacles, whilst another might prefer a green tinge. It's a bit like the ***half-full / half-empty*** syndrome. It is as though we each choose the colour of filter we want to place between ourselves and the external world. Not content with that distortion, our brain then starts to impose a rationalisation process on the incoming information."

Matthew revisited his ideas about left and right. In Latin, French and German, the left was always associated with something sinister or an awkward way of doing something. The right suggested skill. Leaving aside Roman superstitions, there did seem to be something perverse about how the left-brain operated. It seemed always inclined to over-generalise in its efforts to rationalise the irrational. The right, on the other hand – forgive the pun – seemed far more immediate in its processing ability. It seemed to embody the visceral gut-reaction. The left told lies! ***In vino veritas,*** he repeated to himself, realising after last night's alcoholic beverages that the truth will out once inebriation releases the self-imposed constraints of sobriety. Suffice it to say that after this physically created change of perspective, Matthew found himself much more in line with the attitudes of Councillor Williams.

After all, he thought, it is exactly the same world out there that we all experience, so it must be our perception of it that leads us to have such fundamentally different interpretations of it. We see what we want to see. Actually, there is no such thing as external reality: it is always the individual's internal reality that is projected. Those with the most vivid visions control the world.

## Chapter seventeen – the artist

Back in 1980, just to relieve the tedium of the topic for his Master's thesis on ***error analysis***, Matthew had once strayed into parts of the John Rylands Library at Manchester University, not normally accessible to trivial researchers like himself. ***Covert CIA operations in South America***, read the legend on one book spine, and he thought about reviving his earlier career in espionage. Then his eyes settled on what looked like a really fascinating study - Patrick Trevor-Roper: ***The World through blunted Sight***. A cursory glance through the book by this eminent eye-doctor revealed that many artists clearly had – in our terms – defective vision; but that it was this very different way of seeing the world that gave them their artistic talents.

"All art aspires to music," his friend John, (Mr Messy), the artist, once told him. Matthew was in awe of this man who had no compunction about taking on a commission to forge an Old Master, or something more mundane, such as a tax disc, for that matter.
"Surely, it can't be worth the amount of time it would take to reproduce a copy of the original, not to mention having to incorporate all the minor details, as well as acquiring the right inks?" wondered Matthew.
"It's all about the challenge," replied his friend.

Matthew recalled the assistance he had received from Mr "Dizzy" Day, his art teacher at school, in learning how to overlay an original with a grid of squares so that the lines and proportions all matched up. He remembered the other tips Mr Day revealed such as 'looking through half-closed eyes', adding blue to yellow and not vice-versa to make green, getting the right balance when locating abstract shapes on a canvas. Eventually, Matthew reproduced a passable copy of a work he particularly liked, a piece of abstract art by Fernand Leger called ***Les disques***.

Matthew very much appreciated art, but he never really progressed much beyond primary school level, where his class teacher had noted the painstaking way he pursued the task in hand. He felt a connection with his grandmother, Rosa, who preferred oils as her medium of choice, but found himself drawn back to the abstract and the surreal. In later life, computer software packages enabled him to realise his dreams. One eventual design he had generated appealed to him so much that he used it for the CD cover of his 2001 compilation, ***iterative patterns.*** A collection of semi-transparent eggs and stars floated upon a midnight blue firmament. The ovoid beginnings morphed into stellar endings. They seemed to symbolise the processes of birth and death, as he associated with them the mythology behind the naming of the various constellations: Castor and Pollux, for example, the twins that constituted Gemini .

---

Anita had been a remarkably long-suffering wife. When Matthew informed her one day that it was his intention to create the illusion of a square living room out of the existing rectangular room by painting two walls white and two walls black, she just sighed in acquiescence and allowed him to get on with it. His theory had been that white would appear to recede, whilst black would create the illusion of coming forwards. The subsequent obliteration of the black, once he realised how difficult the colour was to live with, had been a much harder task. Another time, Anita let him paint a huge circle in ***Inca Gold*** at one end of the kitchen: at least that looked cheerful, she felt. His ***pièce de résistance*** was to have been the transformation of the - for him – too mundane cuboid living room into a sphere. To achieve this, he had calculated that by using the darkest shades of purple for the eight corners, and the most delicate tints of lilac for the six mid-points located equidistant from floor, ceiling and room-ends, he could create the illusion of living in a bubble. It was probably better for all concerned that Anita drew the line at this flight of fancy, however.

An even more bizarre ***grand design*** was to fail to come to fruition only through lack of available funds: this was the solar-powered phototropic house, which enabled its residents to bathe - assuming the sun was actually shining – in sunlight in the lounge all day long, since the house rotated, almost imperceptibly, faithfully following sunrise to sunset, like the shadow on a sundial, at a speed of 15 degrees per hour, from east to west. Of course, there were some problems with the design: you could not guarantee constant sunshine, and it had to be rotated back to its starting point ready for the next sunrise on the following day.

Nevertheless, Matthew took great pride in his skills as a mere painter and decorator. One long, cold summer back in 1973, he was serving his apprenticeship alongside Jock, painting the railings of a brand-new ten storey car park in Swindon. Matthew had often wondered what the point of school could possibly be for society in general. He vaguely recalled one eminent sociologist (Émile Durkheim) claiming that school should mirror the demands of the world of work. 'At least I got the kids well prepared for this kind of work,' Matthew thought, 'Mind-numbingly boring, repetitive and monotonous tasks like this one. In addition, it could not have been a worse colour of paint: grey. Never mind. At least it inspired one of my jazz compositions.'

***Dazzling grey, never knew a day quite so strong come along.***

***(JS/1973)***

"Don't tell the clerk-of-works;" said Jock, "I'm going to add some spirit to the paint to make it go on more smoothly." Even with this added lubrication, the incessant brush-strokes made it seem increasingly more like a Sisyphean task of Forth Bridge painting proportions.

---

We now move forwards to February in the year 2000. In the hospital, Matthew signed up for everything. There was yoga, badminton, reflexology, relaxation techniques, pottery and art therapy, to name but a few of the options. It was by getting him to commit his daubings to sheets of paper that the therapist got Matthew to explore his inner thoughts. In his picture, the rudiments of a river could be clearly perceived. To the left, where he himself stood, were some less easily identifiable blue and black objects, whilst over the other side of the river was some as yet unattainable green goal. Here he stood, ***alone beside the stream***, as his song had predicted some thirty years before.

When he later took up voluntary work with folk who were experiencing mental illness, he decided to provide his own version of art therapy. Working with empty coffee jars and papier maché, his new-found friends began to ***seize the day***, and he realised that virtually all creative pursuits help to focus the mind on the here-and-now instead of dwelling on past disasters or future fears. Indeed, the very activity, he found, was encouraging his friends to open up and discuss their experiences quite openly, rather than sitting in silence, which is what used to happen.

Matthew remembered that Saint Paul, like many artists, used to have defective vision before he had his conversion to Christianity on the road to Damascus, and resolved to follow in the man's footsteps by taking a pilgrimage to Corinth.

## Chapter eighteen – the pilgrim

In the summer of 1969, learning a few basic phrases of Serbo-Croatian and Greek, before his odyssey that started in Rijeka and finished up in Corinth, came in useful. The twenty-four hour boat-trip to Dubrovnik provided plenty of opportunities to engage with the indigenous population, and the odd ***izvinite, molim*** or ***hvala*** did not go unnoticed. Often it would lead to a conversation in German, if the correspondent had spent some time as a guest-worker in Germany. The coach trip from Dubrovnik to Skopje was similarly entertaining. As people got on the bus with an assortment of chickens, goats and other wild life, local youths took the opportunity to give a rendition of the rebel song, ***Macedonia***, a particularly foolhardy gesture under the regime of Tito, the dictator. It would be like singing ***It's off to Dublin in the green, in the green*** in a predominantly Protestant part of Belfast.

The coach stopped close to Albania for a toilet stop. Seeing nothing more elaborate than a hole in the ground, Matthew followed the old maxim of when in Rome... he had already discovered how to use the unisex facilities of the Rijeka youth hostel standing on one leg with your foot against the door – there being no locks on the doors. He had wondered (since this was to date his only experience of life in a communist country) if privacy was deemed far too bourgeois a luxury. From Skopje, he proceeded to Thessaloniki, Athens and then on to Corinth.

"***Xenon neotitos***?" he enquired, to be greeted only by blank stares. He must have placed the emphasis on the wrong syllables, he thought. Eventually, he found the youth hostel for himself and selected one of the roof spaces, after being alerted to the presence of bed-bugs in the dormitories. Under the generals, Greece was clearly the opposite of a democratic country, but it was remarkably clean with virtually no litter or graffiti, and immaculately tended parks. However, the youth hostel proved to be quite a hot-bed of political debate. The clientele was cosmopolitan and infiltrated by budding terrorists. Anti-Zionist and anti-American literature circulated quite openly amongst the students.

"Why is everyone so anti-American?" asked Matthew.
"Not for the reasons you might assume," replied Hassan, his Egyptian friend. "Everyone is really pissed off with the American Navy. As a good-will gesture, they all donated blood last week. That means now none of us has been able to earn a few drachmas in exchange for a litre of blood. We're all broke and desperately in need of finding a way of making some cash. I really could do with a hair-cut." Matthew took on the challenge of trimming Hassan's ulotrichous locks with relish. He likened the procedure to that of topiary, only on a smaller scale. He used the small pair of scissors that he

carried in his wash-bag. Hassan was most appreciative and wished him well for the rest of his stay.

Coming from a country where getting your hair cut had been the last thing on his mind as a teenager, Matthew had always sported shoulder-length hair whenever he could get away with it, but, paradoxically, he had always been fascinated by the process of cutting hair, enjoying the sensation as he combed out a length, gripped it between his fingers before snipping it neatly away. He prided himself on keeping his father's hair neatly trimmed. He had persuaded his wife to let him cut her fringe, but he never quite got the hang of ***shaping*** women's hair.

The next day, Matthew joined half a dozen assorted nationalities down at the blood donor clinic, feeling a mixture of apprehension and queasiness since this was the first time he had ever given blood.
"Passports, please!" said the nurse. Donors were selected using medically spurious and ethically scandalous criteria: top of the list came white Caucasian Americans; next came Northern Europeans, and Matthew found his name selected; Mediterranean types, including Greeks came next, followed by Arabs and Asians. Blacks, even those from the American Navy, were only selected as a last resort, and Matthew found this ridiculous, since as far as he understood the science, blood types transcended race. "Drink the orange juice, and keep pumping with your arm, suggested the nurse, when he had not given quite the required amount. He had heard horror stories about gullible students being bled dry in less salubrious surroundings, but was soon released with a handful of drachmas to spend on replenishing his perceived drop in blood pressure.

The following day, he headed off to Corinth and was reminded of the constant reminders of Saint Paul in his life. After spending the night on the beach, he awoke to find a regular army of soldier ants disappearing into the distance, carrying away his loaf of bread that he had been saving for breakfast. His thoughts went back to his reading, as an eleven-year-old choirboy, from Saint Paul's epistle to the Corinthians, and how that short message about faith, hope and love had stood the test of time.

## Chapter nineteen – the roofer

Just as shyness can be mistaken for aloofness, so a person with an inferiority complex can project a very superior attitude to the outside world. Matthew's hypersensitivity to any form of criticism projected itself out as a hypercritical treatment of others. Perhaps that is why he so enjoyed this superior location, fifty feet above the ground.

Sometimes, it was just a case of climbing the ladders to the dormer roof before attaching a roof ladder to get him up to the ridge tiles which had worked loose during a storm. He was surprised they had stayed in place so long with just a dollop of cement to attach them. Sitting astride the apex of his house, he would pause to listen out for the distant sounds of church bells, bird-song and children playing. As he ascended and descended the ladders, he would detect the rise in pitch by, perhaps, a semi-tone, of the sounds of the street. The idyll would be periodically interrupted by the blare of a car-horn or the mouth-watering jingle emanating from a passing ice cream van.

Over the years, he became practically an expert in repairs to flat roofs. He would eschew the traditional use of hot pitch to adhere the layers of felt. Instead, he preferred the large drums of the black stuff – there was an element of boyish fun in getting it all over your hands and clothes – and he would always be the lone worker. He realised that teamwork would have got the job done quicker and perhaps with less effort having to lift heavy weights, and run up and down the ladder for the necessary tools, but he had always worked that way. The weight of the drum was such that the base of the ladder sank into his garden soil as far as the first rung. Luckily, the ladder was leaning against the dormer with sufficient spare rungs protruding above the parapet to allow for its partial slide!

Removing the moss was the first exercise, whereupon it became clear that summer heat and winter frosts had stretched and cracked the existing layers. Sometimes he would remove them completely, if he felt that the wooden structure beneath was sound. Otherwise, he would simply trowel on the pitch, making sure that the cracks were well covered before rolling on first the under-felt and then the top layer. Finally, he would complete the 'cake' by adding the icing sugar: white limestone chippings to reflect the sun – a rather unnecessary topping, he felt, given the inclement weather in Manchester.

Matthew had loved clambering up onto roofs from the time when he was a small boy, assisting Mr Elmley, the chimney-sweep (not climbing up inside the chimney, however!). In his dreams, Matthew would frequently return to a familiar house: not one corresponding in any way to one he had actually lived in, but nevertheless the house seemed every bit as real as bricks and mortar. He realised the symbolic significance- the house is usually analogous with the human body and soul - but was his obsession with roofs to do with seeking shelter or merely a subconscious desire to feel superior? He had never experienced vertigo or the ***Peter Pan*** urge when working at heights. He relished the opportunities that roof repairs afforded him to transcend the banal.

Werner, a mental health nurse in Germany, used to say that ***his*** patients suffered from 'roof damage'. Matthew had, in his time, encountered a number of people with psychiatric conditions. He often got incensed when he came across once perfectly ***normal*** individuals reduced to drooling from the side of their mouths and becoming suddenly bloated and obese after being switched quite arbitrarily, so it seemed to him, to the latest pharmacological panacea. The drugs, he maintained, were not therapeutic for the individual: they were a convenient way of sedating some (allegedly) potentially dangerous psychopaths. Very few of the recipients of medication were actually in this category. Often the drugs would exacerbate their problems. Excluding the role ***guinea-pig*** from the equation: what was the point of the medication?

Clearly, there was a financial interest for the drugs companies in expanding their markets, so they were an obvious winner. Doctors received a variety of incentives to prescribe, both directly and indirectly, from the drugs companies, but they had also got used to issuing a prescription, and their patients would feel short-changed if they came away with just a recommendation to sign up for the likes of ***cognitive behavioural therapy.*** Relatives and carers, and especially staff in care homes, found it more convenient, as 'managers', to administer medication rather than actually interact with depressed or distressed persons. The general public liked to imagine life for them was much safer when misfits, eccentrics and maniacs did as they were told and took their medication.

## Chapter twenty – the cook

Analysis, if taken to the nth degree, can lead to disintegration and fragmentation. Analysis is a useful tool, but it needs its opposite, synthesis, to put Humpty-Dumpty back together again. Being able to combine ingredients in the correct proportions to produce a satisfactory conglomerate, be it concrete or a cake, is analogous with the process that represents the defragmentation of the soul.

As all good torturer-trainers will know, sadism has to be nurtured amongst the recruits. Much of the psychology behind the training works on the same principle that we mentioned in connection with the creation of prefects at school. If a recruit displays any sign of humanity, this has to be beaten out of him or otherwise eradicated through psychological means, before he will inflict the pain level required. It could be said that the recruit has to be reduced to the brutalised status of a wild animal before he can be instructed to torture his victims. Yet we know that it is not enough to simply destroy an individual in this way. The would-be torturer has to be rebuilt with a new persona and biography to justify his actions.

It was 1973 and Matthew took on extra work as a labourer for a builder in Slough. As Matthew carefully mixed in the agglomerate in the suggested four parts to two parts of sand and one of cement, he thought how closely the whole process resembled making a cake, though, of course, on a much larger scale. Similarly, as he tried his hand rather unsuccessfully at plastering, having got the initial two layers about right, the final finish was truly like the icing on the cake. Moving on to work as a glazier, Matthew found the manipulation of putty in its linseed oil base much like working with pastry.
"All we need to do now," said Pete, the builder, "is to promote you to accountant, and you can learn how to cook the books, as well!" Matthew never resented the fact that he had had to do so many extra part-time jobs: these sundry apprenticeships ensured that he would later be able to turn his hand to most jobs around the house.

"The army marches on its stomach!" his father had always said, justifying his position as chief cook in the catering corps. Matthew had a sudden image of a battalion of gastropods heading for his prize vegetable patch, and ran outside to sprinkle the garden with slug- pellets. He seriously wondered how the army survived with the limited culinary skills of his father. Having reached his teenage years reared on a rigid regimen of meat and two veg, Matthew was beginning to desire a rather less bland cuisine. His first forays into the exotic were delivered in part thanks to the goddess, ***Vesta.***

Various dried ingredients sprang to life, first as a curry, then later as a paella, chow mien or chop suey. Needless to say, his family refused to try that "foreign muck". Ultimately realising that such pale imitations could not compete with the real McCoy, Matthew started purchasing fresh ingredients, such as coriander, from the local market. In the early days, he would attempt to tickle the palate of his guests with all kinds of oriental spices, the hotter the better, however, he learned to reduce the potency of his dishes after the day he included half a pound of chilli peppers in his ***con carne***. Drinking neat Tabasco from the bottle might have been a safer option for his guests whose heads felt about to explode as they gasped for air and water.

Having stymied the return visit of a whole bus-load of former friends, Matthew agreed to defer to Anita's better judgement in future. After several years out in the cold, the pair were finally rehabilitated into the hospitality circuit as their former victims had either forgotten their ordeal, left the area or inexplicably died! New acquaintances had recently joined their circle of friends and he could count on a certain naivety on their part. Rather surprisingly, Anita and Matthew gained a reputation for cooking excellent meals. Whether it was an Indian Curry, a Russian Stroganoff or an Italian Lasagne, appreciation was evident from the speed with which it disappeared from the plates.

Anita would put her creative talents to excellent use perfecting the puddings. Matthew had once suggested they start up a business called ***Dial-a-Dessert*** which could meet an unfulfilled need in the community. Folks would pass by the cakes counters in the supermarkets, suitably impressed at their will-power in resisting temptation, only later to regret not having purchased a pudding after the main meal did not quite satisfy their appetite. That was the time when a quick call to ***Dial-a-Dessert*** would ensure speedy despatch, rather like that of the pizza delivery service.

Of course, puddings can prove rather difficult to transport, as Matthew discovered once to his cost, when he had prepared a black forest gateau for his German evening class. The cake remained comfortably ensconced on the parcel shelf of his hatchback until he had to do an emergency stop – and it suddenly resembled the one in Richard Harris' MacArthur Park "…***and it took so long to bake it***…". He did manage to salvage most of it, after a little careful re-sculpting.

Though cooking was at one time seen as women's work, today many chefs are male, and the segregation of roles is thankfully no longer so rigidly applied. Similarly, sewing and knitting were at one time the province of women only, but as soon as weaving became mechanised, the men were perfectly happy to claim the profession as their own.

## Chapter twenty-one – the weaver

Are our lives preordained, or do we genuinely have free will? Was Matthew destined to follow in his father's footsteps, working as a weaver in the local carpet factory, (Arthur's brief foray into the culinary world in the army catering corps was abandoned when he resumed civilian life), or could he opt to break the mould and escape his working-class origins?

In 1965, Matthew had been a ***creeler*** at the local carpet factory**.** The job entailed running off wool from one bobbin to another by holding it against the rapidly rotating wheel at the side of the loom. This became necessary whenever they were coming to the end of a carpet run and the weavers did not want to waste new bobbins. The area between the rows of bobbins was claustrophobic and Matthew had to be careful not to walk into the spikes that held the bobbins. (He even traced a phobia he had developed about the spikes piercing his eyes back to those days in the factory). Whenever the creelers took a break, Matthew would discuss the latest popular music with his fellow-workers and occasionally Matthew would bring in the words of a Dylan song. He discovered that Chris Curtis, the drummer with the Searchers, had once worked as a clerk in the offices of the carpet firm. What did the Fates have in store for Matthew? Matthew spent the cash he had earned that summer in the factory on a twelve string guitar, determined to unseal his potential fate. The following year, his earnings paid for a skiing holiday in Innsbruck, and before he left for Austria, he tried out the artificial slope in Rossendale. Strangely enough, the carpet firm he worked for were now manufacturing sections of this artificial ***piste***.

Matthew enjoyed the mythological notion of the Fates weaving our destiny. Clotho span the thread of life, Lachesis measured it and Atropos cut it. The elements of chance and inevitability were integral to the process. Matthew had always liked the work of the Swiss writer, Friedrich Dürrenmatt, and was particularly fascinated by the detailed notes that the author gave about the concept of ***Zufall*** (chance) at the end of his seminal work, ***Die Physiker***, (The Physicists). It seemed like poetic justice when the author died just prior to his forthcoming birthday celebrations that had been so meticulously planned for.

Men's work or women's work? Anita and Matthew had grown up in a world where gender stereotypes had been clearly differentiated from one another. Both had attended single-sex schools and followed the corresponding curriculum. Demarcation disputes rarely materialised in the home as each complimented the duties of the other. However, living through a period where women's liberation was very much on the agenda, Anita had pointed out some of the inequalities in the relationship and insisted that Matthew do more to pull his weight by taking turns at doing the washing, cleaning and gardening, particularly since she was now virtually in full-time work.

They had always taken turns getting up to feed the baby, but now that their children were at school, Matthew did not feel he spent anywhere near enough time with them, especially whilst he was trying to hold down more than one job. He would often do night-shift at weekends, on this occasion either driving taxis or manning the base. Practically simultaneously, he was working on his dissertation and Anita was beginning to resent his not giving her an opportunity to go for her PhD.

Just as Anita and Matthew began to share the tasks around the home, they made a conscious decision not to encourage their son and daughter to limit their options by following traditionally male or female roles, respectively. Matthew taught his son how to weave, whilst Anita taught their daughter how to weld. Whether this led, in its own small way, to a generation with more opportunities to succeed in the world and with more respect for the roles traditionally performed by the opposite sex, or whether it just left them confused about their sexual identity remains to be seen. There was one overriding aim in all of this, however. Unlike in their grandparents' generation, it was hoped that these kids would grow up to be more independent, rather than dependent. In retrospect, it now seems that our society needs to return to a situation where we are ***inter***dependent on one another and less obsessed with every man (and woman) for himself (herself).

"The typing pool used to be exclusively a female domain," said Matthew, "but since the advent of the computer, the lads have taken to keyboarding skills like ducks to water. How did that come about?" Anita remembered how her son had acquired one of the very first home computers whilst he was still at primary school and how he had insisted that she should not come anywhere near his bedroom with the vacuum cleaner in case the magnets damaged the circuitry. She often wondered, thinking of a further example of stereotypes, why girls studied home economics, but it was the men who ended up as top chefs. At least the education department had made some attempt to legitimise what used to be called ***cookery*** by renaming it domestic science. Things were changing for the better, she reflected: even Princess Anne had an HGV licence. "You don't need a bollock to drive a bus!" as the first female driver for Halifax Municipal Transport is alleged to have replied, when challenged by a local male journalist back in 1969 about her suitability for such work.

"Strange how cottage industries start off as women's work, but once they get mechanised it suddenly becomes perfectly acceptable for a man to do the work," said Matthew.
"Give me an example," replied Anita.

"Well, spinning, dyeing and weaving, for example. When I was working with my father in the carpet factory, all the weavers were men. There were women in the factory, but they were kept well away from the men in those days."
"At least we don't get ripped off when we buy carpets," said Anita appreciatively, "You can always pick out the Wiltons and the Axminsters". Matthew thought back to the carpet he had carried back across town to their first home:

***Found a rug***
***In an old junk shop***
***And I brought it home to you***
***Along the way the colors ran***
***The orange bled the blue***

***Paul Simon – I do it for your love***

But that was in their first year of marriage, and ten years later came indications that all was not well between Anita and Matthew.

**Chapter twenty-two – the mourner**

People often react to the end of a relationship in much the same way as they do to a death, but however traumatic either event may be, medication is never the solution. We have to come to terms with such events, and learn, given time, to move on.

In 1982, Matthew soon began to make funeral arrangements on automatic pilot. After his father, his aunt and his boss all died within a period of six weeks, he was starting to believe he was cursed, and when his wife contracted pneumonia and it really was touch-and-go whether she would recover, he adopted "safe mode", shutting down all his emotions and occupying his time rehearsing for a pantomime. To many, this appeared callous, but he put it down to displacement activity.
"The show must go on," he said, but felt really upset when he realised Anita would not be a part of it, as had been planned. Her name appeared in the credits on the programme which had just come back from the printers.

Matthew wished he had been more capable of showing compassion, as he collected Anita from the hospital. True to form, the battery was flat, and the car needed a push start.
"I'm useless," said Matthew, and realised from that moment that Anita would never really be able to love and respect him again. He had tried to reassure his children, but he realised that his young daughter would probably be scarred for life, resigned to the distinct possibility of losing her mother. His son put on a brave face, but Matthew wondered how resilient he was going to be. Fortunately for the children, their mother did survive, but she never quite recovered from the long-term side-effects of the powerful antibiotics she had to take, and she found it hard to forgive Matthew for deserting her in her hour of need.

There was a stillness on the allotment, and Matthew derived great solace there, following his first real encounter with death. Kids were usually shielded from this natural process and told that a relative had gone to heaven, but as a young teenager, Matthew had been staying with his mate, Gary, at a B & B in Scarborough. When Gary's sister could not waken mother, Matthew and Gary had gone to investigate. Matthew knew from the lack of pulse and the bluish colour of her face that the lady was dead. A doctor was summoned, followed by an undertaker and the holiday was over. Matthew lost touch with Gary, but later heard on the grapevine that he had suffered a mental breakdown.

When Anita worked with the terminally ill, she took out a book about the grieving process and Matthew found it comforting, as well as illuminating. He took in the fact that grieving is a natural process that everyone has to go through at some point in their life and regarded it as a rite of passage - just like adolescence or marriage. He felt instinctively that the business of routinely prescribing anti-depressants to the recently bereaved was wrong. From his own limited experience of it, he found medication decidedly unhelpful, prolonging, as it did, rather than accelerating the process of recovery. All the professionals seemed to be saying was, 'stop thinking'. Matthew needed time to think.

## Chapter twenty-three – the walker

Walking, like dreaming, provides an excellent opportunity to think things over.

It was 1968, and one of the highlights of Matthew's hiking escapade was his sojourn at the Neusiedler See, a lake where Austria meets Hungary. He was awakened from his reverie by the sound of storks perched on chimney-pots, and went down to the water's edge to take a dip.
"It's quite healthy," remarked a middle-aged woman, as he emerged like the monster from the swamp, covered in grey mud. The water was quite shallow, probably not much deeper than waist-high across the entire lake. The woman's husband, as it transpired, was yet another émigré, this time from communist Hungary. Lazlo was honoured to meet an Englishman and proceeded to quiz Matthew about the England soccer team who had won the 1966 World Cup. Generally unaccustomed to finding much to be proud of about his nationality, Matthew suddenly rose to the challenge and remembered the rather awkward situation where he and Joachim, a German exchange student, had watched the game together, in a distinctively prickly atmosphere, especially after the disputed goal.

"***You'll never walk alone***..." goes the song, but in Matthew's case, walking had been a very solitary experience. After the previous year's visits to Innsbruck and Salzburg, he decided to set himself the task of walking from Graz to Vienna, a distance of around two hundred miles, where he planned to meet up with Sylvia, his girl-friend at the time. Uncharacteristically for him, Matthew had planned the whole enterprise meticulously, ensuring that he enclosed international reply coupons in letters to each of the youth hostels on the way. He had anticipated that a distance of twenty miles every alternate day would be perfectly adequate and would give him enough time between stops to explore the towns and villages on the way. Dressed somewhat inappropriately by Austrian standards in his customary student attire, Matthew was often taken for a ***Gammler***, but he generally managed to overcome such initial wariness on the part of the locals by communicating with them in German. The one luxury he had afforded himself was a brand new pair of sturdy hiking boots. Inevitably, blisters appeared for the first few days because the boots had not been broken in prior to the trip.

The contrast between the camaraderie in the youth hostels, sharing a beer with students from a variety of nationalities and singing songs to guitar accompaniment, on the one hand, and the splendid isolation on the road could not have been greater. At the one extreme, Matthew really enjoyed having an opportunity to be gregarious and sociable, whilst at the other extreme, he could indulge in one of his favourite pastimes: thinking. He would walk for hours on end without encountering a single soul, content to enjoy communing with nature, as he observed the trees flanking either side of the road which itself continued sometimes, it seemed, interminably into the middle distance. Walking, as he was later to discover, could be extremely therapeutic, and seemed, rather like dreaming, to help resolve the problems of the day.

"I met Vladimir, a Czech dentist, on my travels who had managed to cross the border just before the Russians moved in with their tanks," said Matthew. "He had first gained temporary asylum by marrying a woman from West Germany, but the arrangement didn't work out, so he had to return to Bratislava. That guy, all he had to live on for the two weeks he planned to stay in Austria was the equivalent of about two pounds. He explained to me that since liberalisation under Dubcek, people could travel abroad but were only allowed to exchange that small amount of money."
"There's always someone much worse off than you are," remarked Sylvia, when they finally met up at the ferris-wheel in the Prater, a famous fun-fare in Vienna.
"That's certainly true," replied Matthew. As they took a ride together on the big wheel, Matthew again enjoyed spying down from such a superior position to the streets below, once walked by Harry Lime, the Third Man.

When Matthew reached Wiener Neustadt, he learned that the Youth Hostel had once been the stamping ground of the Nazi Party. He picked up on that intangible, but almost palpable feeling that something evil had happened here. It was as if the very walls of the building had recorded - in some randomly arranged silicon compounds within the stones – the events of yesteryear. He had felt a similar experience in the Dachau concentration camp, but also in the cleared villages of the Scottish Highlands and in Dingle Bay in Ireland.
"Perhaps you're just hypersensitive," concluded Sylvia.
---
When Matthew was put on medication, he found himself joining his fellow zombies in, as it was affectionately referred to, ***the largactyl shuffle***. The restlessness became intolerable. He just could not keep still. Walking was the only way of counteracting the chronic side-effects. At first, these walks were restricted to the grounds of the psychiatric hospital, but later he got allowed out and would generally head off for a couple of hours at a time, sometimes for a walk into the nearby town. On release from the hospital, fearing he would develop tardive dyskinesia, (Parkinson's-like symptoms) if he continued to show "insight" and take the drugs as prescribed, he decided to go ***cold turkey***, and stopped taking all the medication immediately.

## Chapter twenty-four – the servant

***Quis custodiet ipsos custodes?*[13]**

***Juvenal***

It is generally well understood that victims of abuse often return for recurrent bouts of ill-treatment. Similarly, those of us who choose to adopt the role of servant will frequently put up with quite unacceptable levels of abuse from our customers. Inevitably, such pent-up frustration at being on the receiving end of abuse has a habit of flaring up at a later date, in an angry outburst.

Sue followed up her earlier discussion,
"You told me there were many authority figures when you were growing up - the priest, the policeman, the teacher, etc: as an adolescent, how did you challenge their assumed power?" Matthew followed the perfectly normal rites of passage in his teenage years,
"I grew my hair long, explored the opposite sex and had the odd alcoholic beverage." Sue took it one stage further,
"And as an adult?"
"I found it a challenging task to assert my rights, particularly if this meant upsetting the apple-cart. Knowing that I had just as much right to exist as the next man was a lesson that took me years to learn." Sue decided to provoke Matthew, just to see how he reacted,
"So you were a sycophantic, subservient little toad, were you?"

"Like a servant, you mean?" said Matthew, as he began to trace the etymological deterioration of the word, 'servant'. "Everyone's forgotten the true meaning of the word. I'm not advocating that we should revert to treating ***inferior*** people as slaves, like they did in classical times; but look at the nonsensical concepts we face nowadays. Take the 'service industry', for example. Not one of its employees has the slightest intention of providing us with a service: they're more interested in ripping us off! I think the rot set in when restaurants started introducing ***service charges***. And what about so-called 'public servants'? They're only in it for their own advancement, financial or otherwise." Sue noted in her diary: MATTHEW HAS A LOT OF PENT-UP ANGER!

Matthew believed that politics should mirror the roles of minister and server in the church. He began his role as server at Saint Matthew's Church, Lightcliffe, and felt that it had taught him a degree of altruism. He had always found it easier to campaign on others' behalf rather than trying to

---

[13] Who watches the guardians themselves?

advance his own cause. The motto of one of the schools where he had taught had been ***sto ut serviam***[14], and he felt this attitude should be kept firmly in the minds of those whose professions were regarded as vocations as well as those who were elected to represent the interests of their constituents.

As we already know, the bible had been quite influential in the development of Bertolt Brecht, despite his communist credentials, but then Christ would probably have been deemed to have been a fairly good Marxist on the face of things. There was one Brechtian concept that Matthew liked to demonstrate, and that was a kind of role-reversal. The master would become the servant for a day, and the servant the master. Rather than getting the troops to fetch and carry for him, Matthew would encourage them to take centre stage, whilst he would play the runner, the technician, the gofer or even, in some cases, the stooge. He did not like telling other people to do things he was not prepared to do himself. He justified this rather servile work to his superiors (who felt it beneath management to perform such tasks) as leading by example. He could identify with caretakers and cleaners because these had been roles he had seen his own parents perform when he was young. He had observed the often abusive way people in such positions were treated by others of allegedly superior rank.

Matthew had a great deal of time for janitors.
"Why are you lowering yourself to that kind of work?" some of his teaching colleagues used to ask him. Those in the union would complain, "It's a demarcation issue, Matthew. Stick to the job you're qualified to do." Then the health and safety tsar would pipe up,
"We're not insured for you to do this kind of work. What's going to happen if you injure yourself?" But Matthew protested,
"Aren't we supposed to be a team? And don't teams work best when everyone pulls their weight, regardless of the task in hand?" The academics insisted that their role was too important to be undermined by such egalitarian notions. The technicians wanted to preserve their mystique (as well as their jobs) and so they too supported the party line which clearly delineated the roles each employee could and could not perform.

"Why do you have this urge to help the caretakers?" asked Sue.
"Because I feel some empathy for their position," said Matthew. "My father used to look after a church, and I know how much he would have appreciated a helping hand from the congregation. Usually, all he got was a supercilious look from the self-righteous elders who would never have condescended to help him move even a few chairs. Most people just take janitors for granted - until they're ill or go on strike, that is. Managers,

[14] I stand to serve

administrators and workers are all ultimately dispensable as individuals. Someone else can act in a 'caretaker' capacity for them; but no establishment can possibly function without its real caretaker."

"Caretakers are more than just janitors with keys to open the doors," said Matthew. "They are guardians, too, placed in a position of trust with tremendous responsibility. Their role should never be underestimated. And yet, despite this onerous accountability, they are afforded very little authority." Matthew harped back to his arraignment of politicians, "It's quite the reverse for the so-called public servants, the guardians of the State. They have all the authority, but none of the accountability. They have practically usurped the said authority, and they behave pretty irresponsibly. At a more global level, those who have taken it upon themselves to be stewards of the planet neglect the ecological needs of the Earth at their peril – more to the point, putting ***us*** all at peril. Glorified ***bar-stewards***, if you ask me."

Matthew had always questioned why such legislators appeared not to be subject to the very laws they themselves had passed for the benefit of the rest of us, "How come they always get away with it?" he asked. "One of the perks of the job, I suppose. A case of 'do as I say, not as I do', as my driving instructor always used to say." Matthew had become increasingly disillusioned with politicians, "It's getting like a banana republic here," he said, "Politicians used to complain about the degree of corruption amongst politicians in Third World countries. Now, ours are beginning to look just as corrupt. It goes to their heads, the power. Trouble is, once they're in positions of absolute power, it gets increasingly difficult to have them removed, no matter what crime they've committed. Joe Public would have been vilified, incarcerated, and sectioned for far lesser peccadilloes. Notoriety, eccentricity, criminality and megalomania are practically ***de rigueur*** for our guardians of public decency."

"Why do you show such resentment for politicians, Matthew?" asked Sue. Matthew smiled,
"Because they are practically immune from prosecution, and, more importantly, from my point of view, not themselves subject to the draconian powers of detention that exist under mental health legislation, for example," said Matthew. " Have you any idea what it's like when a close family relative is urged to agree to you being sectioned? How could a patient possibly regain the trust that she used to have for that relative? Why do they expect close relatives to connive in the sectioning process?"

Sue wasn't sure.
"It may be the pronouns," she said. If, in your role as a committee member, you were to say '***we*** all think it's a good idea to invite Mrs Jones to the meeting', it would make it harder for individual members of the team to opt

out and say they disagreed. If, on the other hand, the committee member had said ***I*** think…, others would have found dissent more acceptable."

Matthew didn't get it,
"And the connection with having the family in on the sectioning?" he asked. Sue explained,
"It's a form of collective responsibility. That way, it's not solely the doctors who get the blame for the section: the family share that responsibility. And we all know that responsibility shared is responsibility diluted, so the doctor doesn't feel so bad about what she has done. She can console herself with the thought that the relative showed great insight into what were his or her loved one's best interests." Matthew smiled, "Yes, I do feel intense anger towards doctors, too," he concluded.
"Who else is on your hit list?" asked Sue. Matthew had to think.
"Quite a few," he replied, but refrained from identifying them by name.

He had resented the iniquity of a situation which depended on the oppressed being complicit in their own oppression. His father's generation had been taught to grovel before their bosses and those in power, though whether the latter took this behaviour for granted, or interpreted it as sycophancy, they clearly wallowed in the adulation, and valued the respect, or more accurately, the fear that it engendered in their workers. Matthew had nothing against good manners: giving up his seat on the bus to an adult was second nature to him and allowing an elderly or frail individual to go ahead of him in the queue at the Co-op was instinctive, rather than indoctrinated into him by the authorities.

However, women's liberation threw his sense of good manners into disarray. When he held the door open one day for a 'lady' to pass through, as was his wont, the lady turned out to be a 'woman', who made a big thing about the whole charade being demeaning to her gender, so, not surprisingly, the next time he encountered her following him, he really wanted to just let it slam in her face, but thankfully he felt better of the action and insisted she go first,
"After you," he said, maintaining his stance, as he held open the door. She passed through, but with real attitude, glaring at him for treating her as an object.

Matthew remained chiefly a ***provider*** of services as opposed to a ***consumer*** of them. Had the liberated lady heard the way her gender was viewed by the taxi-driving fraternity, no doubt she would have had an apoplectic fit.

**Chapter twenty-five – the taxi-driver**

It was 1981 when Matthew started working on the taxi rank in Bury. The drivers were great fun, with an amazing sense of humour, but they were very much 'old school'. Matthew learned to his cost never to attempt to challenge their prejudices. One day, he casually let slip that he would be cooking his wife a curry that night.
"Nay, lad, you don't keep a dog and bark yourself!" remarked one seasoned chauvinist. And once again, he had to endure the taunts of those with chips on their shoulders about how badly they had been treated by ***teachers***. However, one driver contradicted the others. He had had the pleasure – or otherwise – of attending a school in Rochdale, where Dr Rhodes Boyson had been the Head. (He eventually became a prominent Conservative Minister).
"He were strict, but he were ***fair***," insisted Mick, rolling his r's in a distinctively Ramsbottom accent.

Never underestimate the intellectual prowess of a taxi-driver. They come from a surprisingly wide range of socio-economic groupings. Belinda, Matthew's girl-friend in 1970, made the cardinal error of assuming she could make a joke at the driver's expense by speaking a foreign language that she thought was only understood by her fellow-passengers. When the driver responded in the said language, Belinda was mortified.

Matthew had generally avoided taxis in his younger years, regarding them as a distinct waste of money when he could just as easily walk. He assumed they belonged to a world beyond his means that included such things as five-star hotels, yachts and jets. The limitations of his horizons were quite easily explained: his parents had never owned a house or driven a motor vehicle. Travel by coach and train was common, but the idea of ever taking a plane was unimaginable. Similarly, he had been relatively deprived culturally, so much so that on arriving to complete his studies in London, where everything was on the doorstep, he devoured the Arts with gusto. His working-class upbringing had indoctrinated him with the belief that he deserved to be the ***provider*** of a service, such as taxis, but never the ***beneficiary*** of such a service.

Looking around for some part-time work to supplement his meagre salary as a teacher when he arrived in Manchester, Matthew soon settled on becoming a driver for a private-hire firm. However, he was soon to discover that all was not exactly legitimate about the firm. He should have smelled a rat when he turned up for interview in the owner's kitchen: there was no shop front, and calculating the fares was a rather hit-and-miss operation because the Lada he was given to drive only registered complete miles and not fractions thereof.

"Five pounds, please!" he would estimate, and then judge from the expression on the punter's face whether to reduce or increase the amount.
"Don't you realise who I am?" retorted one cocky little teenager. Matthew had to admit that, since he did not follow football, that particular minor celebrity's stardom had failed to overwhelm him.

Matthew's chances of becoming a chauffeur came to an abrupt end one winter's day, when the Lada's brakes failed and he had no option but to run it into some railings in order to bring it to a halt. Luckily, no other vehicle was involved, so he radioed in to explain and check how he was to report the accident.
"For Christ's sake, don't be involving the police," came the reply, "Anyway, you're sacked!" It transpired that the vehicle had no MOT and the last he heard, it had been spirited away without trace.

In his short time as a driver, he had got to know some of the genuine taxi-drivers, but they explained that getting a licence from the Town Hall would be difficult, not to mention the cost of insurance. Far better, they suggested, would be to work for them as a base operator. It would be ideal for him, because he could fit Friday and Saturday nights around his teaching commitments. The job proved to be less straightforward than he might have assumed. Women usually performed this job, probably because they were so much better at multi-tasking.

On the first Saturday night, all hell broke loose. There were twenty taxis on the rank and they would either wait in line to pick up fares there, or be allocated pre-arranged pick-up points around the town. Once a cab had a fare to a given location, the driver would call in response to a job that Matthew announced over the radio. This turned out to be a bit of a free-for-all, with every driver claiming to be at the scene, though clearly that was impossible. Matthew felt it was like playing cards: he had to remember who had been given which job (much as you try to remember cards played) so that he could arbitrate whenever there was a dispute.

The rank, usually pronounced à la Jonathan Ross, had an intercom and three telephones. There were two distinct ring tones and the third phone had a flashing light. Punters must have wondered what was going on, as they attempted to pass on details, whilst their interlocutor appeared not to be listening – his attention had been drawn to one of the other phones, which (he had been warned) had to be responded to within two rings. Added to these distractions, there were always the customers in the queue outside the door who would periodically bang on the door, requiring reassurance that, yes, a taxi was on its way, and any momentary silence was soon punctuated by messages from the drivers coming in over the intercom.

"Snowdrops on Manchester Road, pass it on," came the coded message that the local police recognised only too well as a warning of a speed trap that the drivers should look out for. Sometimes, drivers were prone to adopt radio silence. The reasons for this were various: occasionally, it was because the female fare was paying ***in kind***; at other times, the drivers would be covering up clandestine affairs that their customers needed kept secret.
"Didn't you realise that we had two fares picking up from the same house within half an hour of each other? You were calmly giving out over the air where Mrs Brown and her fancy-man would be spending the night, blissfully unaware, so it would seem, that another of your drivers had her husband on board!" Such indiscretions Matthew gradually learned to avoid.

'Giving a ride' was often ambiguous on the rank. One night the drivers had competition, but not of the usual private hire variety. As the night wore on, and the queue outside grew longer, would-be passengers started to get frisky. The next time Matthew looked out, the queue had noticeably diminished.
"They've gone off with Vera," said one of the remaining punters.
"Hurry up, lads, you've got competition!" urged Matthew. The following week, his next-door neighbour, a policeman who happened to be doing a stint on vice-squad, confirmed that they had picked up Vera that night.
"They must have been pretty desperate," he said, "she was - in my estimation – well into her fifties, wore an overcoat and little else underneath, but what I think would have turned most people off, she had left her false teeth at home." They did not keep policemen on vice squad for too long in case it corrupted their own already warped minds. Peering down through strategically placed spy-holes in the public conveniences at a local Justice of the Peace who has an assignation with one of the local rent-boys cannot be good for the soul, over the long term.

The thing about taxi-drivers is their reputation for straight-talking. Delivered in the 'restricted code' it may well be, but they do come straight to the point. They call a spade a bloody shovel, as his father might have said. Matthew soon began to realise that having a million word vocabulary does not mean that you will be any more concise in your efforts to communicate, and some would say that it is the very use of the so-called 'elaborated code'[15] that impedes communication.

[15] Basil Bernstein, 1971

# *Episode II*

## Chapter twenty-six – the etymologist

**In the beginning was the Word, and the Word was with God; and the Word was God**

**The Gospel according to Saint John, Chapter 1**

As a keen etymologist, when his life started to disintegrate, and as the millennium approached, Matthew started searching for meaning.
"The gift of language," said Matthew, "seems to mark us out as somehow different from all other species on the Earth, and it would seem that every generation has tried to trace back the original meaning of words since time immemorial. This appears to run parallel to our interest in genealogy, since, in tracing our family histories, we are trying to connect with our forebears. We all have the desire to leave some trace of ourselves to future generations, even if it is just the creation of children, and we crave immortality just as we admire celebrity, because we vainly hold on to the hope that we might be remembered in years to come for some good deed we performed, some piece of music we composed, some battle we won, some edifice we constructed, some work of art we created, or some book we wrote."

"Why are you looking for meaning in the past?" asked Alice. "It's the here and now that's important. Remember what David Crystal says about the usage of words. It's what they come to mean through current usage, not what they originally meant." "***Wicked!***" retorted Matthew, emulating the vernacular. "See! That's yet another example of etymological amelioration."
"But don't forget the power of the etymology of the people," said Alice, "Particularly with all the amateur researchers on the internet, soon we'll all be communicating in text-speak, you mark my words!"
"As I was saying," said Matthew, "before you all got me off on another tack altogether, mankind has always tried to identify the origins of words. Take Vergil, the Roman writer, for instance. He surmised that the reason why Lake Avernus had got its name was down to its derivation from Greek, meaning there were no birds [cf: ornithology] in its vicinity."

"You could, of course, go back to biblical times," said Alice. "Golgotha is translated for us in the bible as ***the place of the skull*** and it's possible that Jesus himself used the word, as he is assumed to have spoken Aramaic."
"So what did ***mene, mene, tekel, upharsin*** mean, do you think?" said Matthew.
"That was the writing on the wall in the book of Daniel," said Alice, "Maybe a warning then, but perhaps, even more significantly, a warning to us, now. Money and shekels relate to the first two expressions. Think of our use of the pound as a unit of currency. Usually, the explanation goes

something like this: 'you have been weighed in the balance and found wanting. As a punishment, all your possessions will be divided up amongst the Medes and Persians."
"And today," said Matthew, "what's the great significance of the writing on the wall? Is it just Hebrew graffiti?"

"Remember that movie we saw together, ***Double Indemnity***, I thought one of the best lines was the one that went something like this: 'Money is like manure: it's absolutely of no use unless it's spread around a bit.'
"If I remember correctly," said Alice, "dreaming about excrement is supposed to signify your attitude towards money, so the two are clearly related." Alice continued, "It could apply to the current financial crash, don't you think?" Matthew felt the anger welling up inside him.
"All those bankers, gambling now with money lent to them by the government (i.e. taxpayers' money) so they can carry on gambling, risk-free. Once they've lost their bail-out money, they can claim it on insurance, which the government (i.e. the taxpayer) has agreed to underwrite. About time more of the Western billionaires started to make some philanthropic gestures, if you ask me, otherwise Daniel's prophesy might come true, and they'll see their fortunes confiscated and redistributed to the Third World, the present-day equivalent of the Medes and Persians. The prophesy resembles a numerological conundrum that needs an etymologist to choose the correct translation. Do we use the term 'divide' or do we use the term 'share'? A semantic nuance, you may protest, but think of the implications of these two words from a political standpoint. ***'Divide and conquer'*** is a policy for subjugating the masses, whilst ***sharing*** is designed to be for the common good."

"Why not trace language back to the Tower of Babel, in that case?" suggested Alice, "Perhaps most languages do emanate from the same source, after all, we can see how early languages thrived, only eventually to be subsumed and replaced by newer languages. That was certainly the case with Latin and its romance language derivatives. Where do you reckon they all came from?" Matthew pondered for a while, recollecting his earlier studies.
"Probably Sanskrit's the furthest back we can go, I remember one category of expressions that was called ***bahuvrihi compounds***. Literally, the expression means a lot of rice, but it actually referred to a ***person*** who had a lot of rice, i.e. a rich man. Fascinating stuff, isn't it?"

Alice's silence spoke volumes. She was secretly worried about the destructive effect that all this 'thinking about thinking' could have. Much of the initial research into reflection and metacognition was associated with obscure religious sects whose sole interest was in controlling the minds of their converts. Having destroyed their victims through extreme analysis, they could rebuild them as compliant believers. She was later to observe the virtual disintegration of Matthew and wondered how he would ever be able to put himself back together again.

## Chapter twenty-seven – the analyst of the spirit

When Matthew reached the very depths of his subconscious mind, after he had dipped into reminiscences he had assumed were long ago extinct, in a state of hyper-arousal where the surreal was infinitely more tangible than the virtual reality of everyday existence, he finally felt well-and-truly lost, down a system of roads without signposts. It was at this nadir in the year 2000 in the middle of the night in his rented flat that his spirit guide, Jean-Paul, appeared to him.

"Look into the mirror," said Jean-Paul, "What do you see?" Matthew hesitated.
"My reflection?" he ventured.
"Look closer," suggested Jean-Paul, "Scry more deeply into the well." A couple of minutes passed, then Jean-Paul continued, "Now let's take away the mirror. What image do you ***remember*** seeing?" Matthew was perplexed.
"Nothing, to be perfectly frank. I could lie, of course, and give you the perfectly reasonable answer that it was image of my face, but that's only because I know that that is what I ***expect*** to see when I look into the mirror."

"That's good, now we're getting somewhere," said Jean-Paul, "Now smash the mirror, go on, hit it with the hammer!" Matthew was reluctant to comply with this instruction, fearing it would lead to seven more years of hard luck stories, but he eventually relented, and was immediately fascinated by the effect, like a child playing with a kaleidoscope for the very first time. "Now look into the mirror. What do you see?" asked Jean-Paul.
"A distorted reflection," replied Matthew.
"Come on, use your imagination," urged Jean-Paul.
"A myriad of tiny reflections of parts of me," replied Matthew.
"And that's a true reflection of the schizophrenic mind," explained Jean-Paul, "So having symbolically recreated a reflection of your condition, we're now going to set about reversing the process."

"However can you do that?" asked Matthew. "I've never seen anyone capable of re-assembling all the shards of glass and then somehow fusing them back together again."
"Rewind the video-tape," said Jean-Paul. Matthew watched as the tiny smithereens reunited to restore the mirror to its pristine condition.
"I see: it's like my glasses," said Matthew, "however much I twist them and distort them, they always return to their original shape – apparently memory is built into them."
"Well, we wouldn't want you getting a distorted view of the world, now would we?" said Jean-Paul, with a wry smile.

"Remember," said Jean-Paul, "Try to put like with like: everything has got jumbled up in your head. That's why you've got all your expletives confused. And the very fact that you don't very often actually come out with swear-words means they're bubbling away subliminally, festering beneath the threshold of the conscious mind, infecting your thinking. Once you begin to tell the difference between excrement and treasure, you'll be ready to make a start."
"So, you're saying that I'm a little indiscriminate, are you?" asked Matthew.
"A little?" scoffed Jean-Paul. "To use the vernacular, you don't know your arse from your elbow!"
"That's a bit derogatory," said Matthew. "Where's your evidence?"

"Let's start with the obvious," said Jean-Paul. "A letter arrives, what do you do with it, once you've opened it and read the contents: file it or bin it?" Matthew took his time, carefully recalling his usual routine.
"I put it in the pending tray," he said.
"That wasn't one of the options," said Jean-Paul, "but please explain why you do that."
"Well, I can't throw it away," said Matthew. I may later need it for evidence."
"So why don't you file it, if you think it's so important?" asked Jean-Paul.
"I wouldn't have a clue under which category to file it," said Matthew.

"Precisely," said Jean-Paul. "And that's why you've got such a chaotic filing system in your head. Everything is stored under ***pending*** in the hope that by procrastinating any decision-making on your part your brain will somehow eventually assimilate or accommodate the raw, unprocessed data. Even the way you arrange your folders on the computer speaks volumes. How can you ever retrieve a file if you don't have an appropriate umbrella concept for it? Subsumption doesn't work like osmosis, you know."

"You remember the office maxim: 'you should only ever touch a document once'? By implication, that means that if you don't heed this advice, you will waste an inordinate amount of time searching through reams of paper in a vain attempt to find information. Until you put some order into your physical clutter, there's no hope of you de-cluttering your thought processes. You'll never be a scientist until you can make one simple decision: is it ***yes*** or is it ***no***? Remember, most artistic people have a problem with this; they always hunt for shades of grey, when the answer is either black or white, so don't fall into that trap, at least not in this instance. Now you must forgive me, but it's time to don my philosopher's hat."

## Chapter twenty-eight – the confidante

Jean-Paul had started to appear to him back in November, but Matthew instinctively knew to keep quiet about such visitations. He continued to indulge in regular meetings with Alice, who valued their frank exchange of opinions. Like most men, Matthew did not really have male colleagues whom he could trust to be his confidants. The relationship with Alice, on the other hand, was ideal, and Matthew hoped that Alice would see it as a mutually advantageous arrangement.

Usually Matthew had been quite good at coping with stress. Doctor Martin, his G.P., was to point out that he clearly needed more, rather than less stress in his life. At the time, he found this an odd remark, but came to understand its significance once he took on a job with far greater responsibilities than he had ever had previously.
"The thing about stress, "said Matthew, "is that it has a lot to do with control, as do so many aspects of our lives." Alice wanted to compare notes with Matthew, who had been promoted about the same time as her to Head of Department.
"How did you respond to the increased responsibility?" she asked.

"When you're actually in charge of a department, it doesn't matter how great the challenge is. Since I can personally determine how tasks are to be completed either by myself or, in delegated form, by others, there is no real stress, because the tasks are not generally being imposed by others on me. As I have a personal stake in the outcomes, I actually enjoy the challenges much more. In the past, I could always blame the manager, if things went pear-shaped and console myself with the fact that it wasn't my crackpot scheme in the first place. Those with an inferiority complex have a tendency to shift the blame onto others, just in the interests of self-preservation. Now, I don't need to pass the buck; I can willingly acknowledge the fact, if the failure is my responsibility. If I am under stress, it's good stress."

All went well in the new job, until a situation arose that was totally out of Matthew's control, and management appeared to be looking for a scapegoat.
"Be careful how you use that intellect of yours," said Alice, "remember what Godfrey always says, ***no one likes a smart-arse***." Matthew realised he had won a number of verbal battles hands-down, but he did not want these to become Pyrrhic victories, where the consequential loss far outweighed the gain. Alice had been on the receiving end of retribution herself, having raised her head above the parapet once too often. "It's all about paying you back, don't lower your guard for one minute, you don't need to be paranoid to realise they're out to get you!"

Sure enough, Matthew found himself summoned to a meeting which seemed, on the face of it, perfectly innocuous. It was all about some new initiative about which he had shown himself to be somewhat less than enthusiastic. Very soon, he realised he was in some kind of kangaroo court with accusations being hurled at him left, right and centre. It was then that future advice from his spirit guide might have come in useful.
"Remember, Matthew," Jean-Paul was to counsel, "truth is a very powerful weapon. If you use it judiciously, you can demolish the opposition, regardless of the size of their army of sycophants, even if they've all rehearsed their scripts. To sing effectively from the same hymn sheet, the anthem itself must be worthy: if not, all they'll end up with is a cacophonous catalogue of calumny. Tell the truth and shame the devil."
Like many autistic individuals, Matthew failed to grasp the social necessity for lying under certain circumstances, or at the very least, maintaining his right to remain silent. This is, after all, how all courts function, kangaroo or otherwise. The upshot was that Matthew was threatened with disciplinary action for dereliction of duty.

Although he came away from the meeting feeling vindicated, the whole experience had taken its toll on his sanity. People whom he had numbered amongst his friends had either colluded in his character-assassination by echoing the management line or given their tacit approval of his condemnation by not attempting in any way to help to exonerate him from blame. He stayed up that night, listing the names of his colleagues and devising a shorthand that consisted of brackets and other punctuation marks to indicate their level of trustworthiness[16]. Individuals with three exclamation marks after their names were clearly to be avoided; question marks urged caution and brackets implied total integrity. His mistake was to share this information with management, which, had he been acting rationally, he never would have done, of course. In fact, this very communication precipitated his propulsion into a six month 'holiday' from work. Ironically, however, the sojourn felt more like being exiled to Siberia.

Realising he might shortly be sectioned, given his aberrant behaviour patterns, Matthew resolved to abscond, taking the early train. Train travel would now prove difficult, whether it was at times of hypomania or under the zombiefying influence of prescribed medication. In the former situation, he could not resist conversing with his fellow-passengers, much to their alarm, whilst in the latter case, an attack of the screaming habdabs, or whatever you want to call it, was hard to control because he had nowhere to escape to. The best option was to use the corridors for extensive walking therapy, or the toilets to regain composure. It was the sheer endlessness of the tedious twelve-hour journey that suddenly became unbearable. Under

---

[16] See appendix (ii)

normal circumstances, he would have taken the time to read a novel, or ***in extremis*** doze off, perhaps.

He was sufficiently ***compos mentis*** to write a letter to Alice by way of explanation for his sudden departure so that they did not send out a search party for him. Anita had arranged to meet him at the other end, which was fortunate, because his strange charismatic glow had clearly attracted the attention of the authorities. A contingent of policemen was looking menacingly in his direction as he disembarked from the train.

Matthew, despite having socialised with a number of friends from the police ***service*** (note the subtle change from police 'force'), was still in awe of these authority figures whose very uniforms were enough to aggravate his mania. It came as a great relief to him to discover that the investigating officer was an old friend. This was mutually advantageous, because it meant that Matthew was less reluctant to reveal his thoughts and feelings than he would have been with a total stranger. Andy was the avuncular kind of individual whom villains both respected and hated at the same time. Like the taxi-driver's headmaster, he was firm but fair. Teenage delinquents referred to him as ***Robocop***. He had a great sense of humour and the natural authority that is gained after years spent in the armed forces. Yet his authority was deserved, not assumed.

## Chapter twenty-nine – the detective

"You know what they say about schizophrenia?" said Andy who was just about to embark on a course in offender profiling.
"I assume," said Matthew, "that you're about to tell me one of the many jokes proliferating from this fertile breeding ground?" Andy shook his head.
"No. For once, in the immortal words of our classic jazz trumpeter, Steve, ***'I'm not trying to be funny'.*** I think you'll find this conclusion intriguing, given your obsession with words."
"Go ahead, then," said Matthew, "Spill the beans!" Andy was very good at timing, unlike Matthew who would always seem to either misread the cues from his interlocutors or end up interrupting the direction the conversation was going by interjecting an apparent non-sequitur. This was the reason why Andy was much better at delivering jokes than Matthew.
"It's the way I tell them," quipped Andy in a close parody of Frank Carson.

"That reminds me of the joke about the Trappist Monks," said Matthew. "A novice joins the order one day and witnesses a form of group therapy going on, using humour as the essential ingredient. The novice receives his copy of the ***ninety-nine best jokes*** book. As we all know, Trappist monks are not allowed to speak, and so each monk in turn was holding up one or two cards with numbers printed on them. 'Does this happen regularly?" asked the novice, momentarily forgetting his vow of silence. To this blatant infringement of the rules the abbot held up a huge card with the letters SHH! inscribed upon it. Duly admonished, the novice sat out the remainder of the session, observing smiles, accompanied by muffled bursts of laughter, as successive sets of numbers were held up for all the group to see. Most of the monks seemed familiar with the code since they smiled instantaneously on seeing a given number, whilst others had to leaf through the small decoding booklet before they got the joke. After the session, the novice was curious and wrote down his question hoping his mentor would explain: 'It doesn't seem to matter which set of numbers is held up, it's only Francis who produces hilarity amongst the entire group.' The mentor scribbled his response, 'It's the way he tells them!'

Andy cut straight to the chase:
"Schizophrenia is the price we pay for our ability to use language." Matthew pondered this pronouncement,
"In the grand scheme of things, probably a price well worth paying," he said.
"I have heard there's a statistically significant correlation between schizophrenia and bilingualism," said Andy, "though that might include immigrants who have psychologically separated their native tongue for their emotional self from their second language which they've reserved for their

intellectual self – you know, kids that associate English with school and Bengali with home and family, for example."

Andy wanted to discover more about Matthew,
"Are you bilingual, Matthew?" he asked.
"Strictly speaking, no. I didn't start learning German till I was fifteen, by which time most of my neural networks had all been well established; particularly important is the ability of the ear to discriminate new sounds which, by the time I reached fifteen, would have practically disappeared. Even so, I was able to pass myself off as a German in some parts of Austria."
"Would you say that you compartmentalised emotional language separately from your intellectual language?" asked Andy.
"The distinction for me was quite different," said Matthew. "The German language enabled me to be someone with far more authority than I would ever enjoyed within my English persona. It's a very ***masculine*** language, in my humble opinion." Andy smiled.
"Why do you say that?" he asked.
"It sounds masculine, for a start, and my ***alter ego***, my car, is ***der Wagen***, none of your ***la voiture*** or ***la macchina***; even the English think a car is female, for Christ's sake!" said Matthew.
"So it seems to be the opposite way round with you, as far as the emotional and intellectual self are concerned," said Andy.

"Not exactly," replied Matthew. "You see, I never really possessed an emotional vocabulary; both my identities, English and German, were intellectual."
"So you were all head and no heart?" concluded Andy.
"I suppose so," admitted Matthew, "both German and English acquaintances commented on the fact that I never swore and more significantly, perhaps, that I never used any exclamatory expressions in my everyday speech. This fact, accompanied by my 'dead-pan' facial expression led many people to conclude that I didn't care about some traumatic event in their lives simply because I just didn't appear to react in any way."

Andy wanted to check out as many avenues as possibly, and he knew Matthew would be cooperative in this process.
"Let's start with your birth," he began, "was it a difficult labour for your mother, especially at her advanced age?"
"I know I was a forceps delivery, and that I weighed nine pounds. I think I might have been overdue. Bearing in mind that my mother was always rather emaciated at around only eight stones in weight, it's probably a miracle that either of us survived," said Matthew.
"So there may have been some brain damage attributable to the forceps delivery, or deprivation of oxygen," noted Andy.

He then turned to the RTA.
"You mentioned feeling different after the head injuries," he said, "could you elaborate, please?" Matthew tried to recall the changes that had taken place some fifty years before. 'Climb every mountain, till you find your dream', went one song of the day, and Matthew always knew that the life ahead of him would be challenging; not necessarily physically challenging, more mentally challenging – a ***manic mountain***, no less. The road traffic accident had left him with a fractured skull at the age of seven. Strangely enough, it was just after this incident that his intellect kicked in. Later on, he read - as an adult - with some concern, about the increased chances of developing mental illness in people who had suffered such trauma to the head as a child, and was constantly on the alert for apparent changes in his personality.

"I suddenly felt – with hindsight I can put it into words – motivated to succeed, and from then on, I felt I was determined to escape my working class origins and aspire, though to what, at that stage, I was still unsure." Andy prompted Matthew with a reminder of the usual symptoms associated with trauma to the head,
"Would you say you were ever neurotic?"
"That's for others to judge," said Matthew, "though I once did one of those surveys which flagged me up as quite neurotic."

"And did you ever exhibit violent tendencies?" asked Andy.
"That depends on your definition of ***violent***," said Matthew, "my violent outbursts were generally restricted to a slap across someone's face: nothing that would leave a permanent scar – just a response that would trigger maximum humiliation in return for minimal physical effort on my part." Andy appeared concerned,
"And who was this violence directed towards?" he asked.
"I suppose ***you*** would think it was against poor defenceless women and children?" asked Matthew, anticipating Andy's suspicions.
"Let's take it one step further," suggested Andy. "Did your violence ever go beyond the odd slap?" Matthew hesitated. Honesty needed tempering with discretion.
"If you mean the use of weapons or other blunt implements, no; though I might have resorted to giving the odd deserving male victim a good kicking from time to time, though never to the head, of course."

"And did you enjoy that experience?" asked Andy.
"Not particularly, no," replied Matthew. "It felt like I'd failed. A person like me with vocabulary that could intimidate some real villains should have been better able to control his temper, and since the violence was meted out to opponents who were weaker than myself, I found that whole ***Mein Kampf*** excuse rather spurious. I like to think that I can generally adhere to

my old school motto, ***doctrina fortior armis***[17], in discovering how to win arguments and ultimately battles through the careful selection of words."

Andy saved his most telling question till last.
"Did you finally find a worthy adversary on whom to vent your spleen?" Matthew nodded,
"Yes, I did. He was a hard man from Salford, and though he was tooled up, unlike myself, I felt I was able to give as good as I got." Andy was intrigued,
"How did you feel after the encounter?" Matthew smiled as he recollected the feeling approaching what he understood to be euphoria,
"Exhilarated!" he replied.
"Nice to know you are capable of showing your emotions," said Andy, "but have you found some way of keeping these potentially violent outbursts in check, or some way of sublimating them, to some extent?"

Matthew explained his motto,
"***Creative, recreative or procreative***: that's the solution."
"Do please explain," begged Andy.
"My potentially violent outbursts can be spirited away, or at the very least be contained by indulging any one of these three passions. In the creative domain, I can thrash away on my electric guitar at full volume in the garage, or compose a few lines of prose on the computer; in the recreative sphere, I can lift weights, walk, cycle or swim; and finally, provided I have a willing partner – and I would never condone rape, including rape within marriage – there's always sex." Andy seemed satisfied,
"It seems like you've got your condition well under control now," he concluded.

"Aren't you going to probe my sexual fantasies to decide whether they're normal or abnormal?" asked Matthew.
"You'd be surprised what counts as ***normal*** in that area," replied Andy. "You might be surprised to hear that some women imagine 'entertaining' a whole army of men: it's not just a male preserve to fantasise about three-in-a-bed romps. What happens within the privacy of consenting adults' homes shouldn't concern the police, provided no one is likely to get hurt, either physically or mentally."

Matthew wanted to find out how the police service reacted to exhibitionism.
"Obviously, there are situations where you have to intervene for the sake of public decency, but where do you draw the line?" asked Matthew.
"Anyone caught ***in flagrante delictu*** in a public place, such as on a beach, could theoretically be prosecuted. Not only that, but they might end up on

---

[17] The pen is mightier than the sword

the sex offenders' register, depending on the outrageousness of the crime," said Andy.
"I've heard of folk ending up on the register for just taking a leak," said Matthew, "though as far as I'm aware, only men have been targeted." Andy corrected him, "The law affects women and men on an equal basis," he said, "quite often, however, today's ***ladettes***, tanked up on God knows how many pints, usually end up getting charged with a breach of the peace."

"So what's an abnormal fantasy?" asked Matthew, returning to topic.
"As any sex therapist worth his or her salt will tell you," said Andy, "a healthy fantasy can really spice up your relationship, leading to greater arousal and fulfilment: it's just a means to an end, provided it's confined to the relationship in question; and don't forget, it's good to talk with your partner about these fantasies, provided she's prepared to self-disclose too."

Matthew was reluctant to divulge his inner secrets just like that for fear of destroying the relationship by having admitted to some perceived perversion that his partner didn't regard as normal.
"I take it, you have to go easy on things like cross-dressing and fetishes about shoes?" he ventured.
"I wouldn't dream of revealing anything like that, if I were you, unless she expressed an indication of similar propensities," said Andy, "Once the fantasy distances you from your partner, it's time to get worried. Sexual experiences focussing on objects, animals, voyeurism and certain exhibitionist traits are a sign that all is not well. This may vary for gay couples, of course; there's no hard and fast rule."
---
"Oral sex?" screamed Mrs Gorsky to her husband, "Oral sex? Whatever are you thinking of? The day you get to have oral sex with me will be the day that kid next door walks on the moon!" Unfortunately, or fortunately (who can imagine how it panned out?) for Mrs Gorsky, that kid next door turned out to be Buzz Aldrin. Pentagon sources were very perplexed when Buzz allegedly said approximately the following words: 'Good luck, Mr Gorsky!' as he walked on the surface of the moon. They thought it might be a covert message to the Russians!

## Chapter thirty – the accused

For the first couple of months of the year 2000, Matthew had recurrent dreams where the scenario was the law court. We shall hopefully see how characters from the legal system began to figure in Matthew's life, and how he began to find it increasingly difficult to work out whether they were real people in the real world or imaginary characters in a fantasy world. That discrimination is harder to distinguish than you might think. One might assume that time and place should have given him a clue, perhaps? If he was in bed, and it was night-time, you would imagine that he would eventually wake up from the nightmare and realise he had only been dreaming; if it were during daylight hours, and he was in town, he ought safely to assume this was reality? Unfortunately, when madness takes over, all distinctions between reality and fantasy start to blur. You inhabit a world where it is permanently twilight and you cannot differentiate at all.

Matthew felt, in these dreams, that he was on trial for a crime, the nature of which he was unaware, with an indeterminate sentence ahead of him. His very integrity was at stake. If he answered the Judge's questions wrongly, despite not understanding their purpose, he would be condemning himself; he would literally disintegrate. The ceiling in his bedroom had been decorated for its previous occupant, a young girl. There was a pattern of stars above his head that reinforced the idea that he was in cloud cuckoo land.

The accused stood in the dock. He was met by a barrage of questions from the prosecution and the judge who seemed to have decided on a guilty verdict already. "You see, Matthew," said Elaine, his barrister, a person of undoubted integrity, "You're being tried for a crime you're ***going to*** commit. It's rather like the confessions that assassins used to make prior to their deadly deeds. I don't understand for the life of me how the Catholics manage to get so guilt-ridden when they can get off with three Hail Mary's when they go to confession. I thought the penance was supposed to atone for the crime."

"You'd be surprised," said Matthew, "how many Catholic women were in the psychiatric hospital at the same time as me, suffering from schizophrenia and the like. Every so often, there would come an eruption of religious zealotry, peppered with unmentionable expletives emanating from some sweet young lady with whom you'd been having a perfectly rational conversation minutes before. I put it down to the religious leaders not taking on board their ***Piaget.*** Seems to me that the Jesuits have got you by the time you're seven, so there's little chance of you developing without being plagued by images of hell and damnation from then on, and I can't

see how the poor kids can take in all those abstract concepts at such an early age.
"How can you tell that the patients are starting to hear voices?" asked Elaine.

"Sometimes they'll start chuntering to themselves, sub-vocalising in a hushed whisper. It's hardly surprising that they're prone to hearing voices – it used to happen regularly in biblical times, only then most folk were religious and so accepted the messages as coming from God - as well as from somewhat less divine figures - as perfectly normal. Now that the majority of us are agnostics (since we can't be bothered to come out as atheists), the psychiatrists have taken over the role that the priests used to perform, and they've no interest in acknowledging the possibility that hearing voices could be a gift. After all, even today, in what we euphemistically call the 'developing world', those who hear voices are celebrated as shamans. Perhaps, not surprisingly, the incidence of mental illness in such cultures is at a much lower level than the current one-in-four diagnosed in the western world. They wouldn't be able to pay the exorbitant amounts of money for the medication, in any case. Poverty can sometimes be a blessing in disguise."

"That is all very interesting," said the Judge, "but hardly relevant to your crime. Since your crime will be committed in the future, I don't suppose you'll be giving us your alibi? After all, if you don't know ***where*** it takes place, you can't claim to have been somewhere else or with someone you are perhaps yet to meet. Now what's your motive going to be, let me see, ***Covetousness***? – No, we never could get you on that one. They say every man has his price, but you're just not interested in money or possessions. ***Gluttony***? – Obviously not, judging by your emaciated appearance. ***Sloth***? – No, you're a workaholic. ***Envy***? – Can't accuse you of that, either. ***Pride***? – Nothing much to be proud of, have you? ***Lust***? – I think we can let you off with the handful of minor affairs you've had. I can't possibly blame you for something I regularly engage in myself - just for light relief, of course: this job's very taxing, you know."

"That leaves ***anger***, doesn't it?" asked Matthew. I thought that was one of the natural phases everybody goes through when they're trying to resolve traumatic events that happened in their lives?" The judge selected a literary reference for his next diatribe. "You're an ***angry old man***; your ***magnum opus*** will be entitled, 'Look ***forward*** in Anger'. So, spill the beans, what are you angry about?"
"What have you got?" asked Matthew, suddenly taking on the persona of the ***rebel without a cause***. "There are plenty of things in my life I could – with justification - feel angry about, but I don't usually resort to violence - I think I'd enjoy the adrenalin rush too much, and I might get used to that."

"Like when you used to organise the punch-ups on the football terraces?" prompted the judge, "Or that time when you, the wounded warriors, came back to Mike's party, immediately triggering the admiration of the assembled guests for helping to chase off the gate-crashers?" Matthew relished the memory.
"Now that truly was something special," he mused.

"The worst thing about you quiet individuals," said the judge, "is your unpredictability. You put on that calm exterior whilst inside the volcano's ready to blow its top at any second. There are no warning signs, like minor tremors, for example. It's like your handler has used post-hypnotic suggestion to implant a trigger- word on the hearing of which you will carry out the hit. It's not healthy, suppressing all that anger. Of course, unlike the rest of us, you don't know who the victim is going to be, do you?"
"No idea," said Matthew, "can't you give me a clue?"
"Well, I can tell you it's someone you know very well," said the judge. "Actually, there will be multiple victims."

Matthew wondered who the victims might be. What were the flaws in their characters that made them fair game for extermination? He needed to consult his ***operis personae***[18]. But first he would need to learn how to sort the wheat from the chaff, and it was Jean-Paul who again came to his rescue.

---

[18] See operis personae, page 9

## Chapter thirty-one – the Spiritual Philosopher

Jean-Paul reappeared this time in the guise of Michelangelo's Philosopher, significantly dressed in shades of grey and brown, rather than black and white.

"So now you're the ***lover of wisdom***, are you?" Matthew asked his spirit-guide. "What kind of philosopher are you, Jean-Paul? Perhaps the kind who ***stoically*** accepts his lot, saying something like, 'c'est la vie', when traumatic events turn your world upside down. Or maybe you're the medieval kind of philosopher who dabbles in the occult world of alchemy, epitomised in the concept of the ***philosophers' stone***. Or Diogenes, now he was a barrel of laughs, wasn't he?"
"No need to be flippant," chided Jean-Paul, "it's an honourable profession that has had an amazing impact on the world, when you consider it, and I don't just mean the Greeks like Aristotle and Plato: don't forget the impact, far beyond China, of Confucius, who was around in 500 BC; or al-Farabi, the tenth century Muslim polymath from Persia, or Sankara, the Indian philosopher who explored ideas about the self in the eighth century. In recent times, we have witnessed a proliferation of German philosophers..."
"Yes," interrupted Matthew, "I like the German ***Weltanschauung***. I remember buying German translations of the works of Aristotle, because they were unambiguous as compared to their equivalents in English."
"Perhaps you should have read them in the original Greek," remarked Jean-Paul.

"Hang on, you're not Sartre, are you, not sure if I can take all that existentialist crap," said Matthew. Tactfully ignoring this comment, Jean-Paul continued,
"Just as some folk argue anachronistically that Christ was a Marxist, you could make out an equally good case for Christ being an existentialist," said Jean-Paul. "Look at his use of parables. It's a way of getting his audience to reflect. Ultimately, the moral choice in the matter is handed back to them."
"Sounds to me," said Matthew, "like we're back to psychosexual development." "Excuse me," said Jean-Paul, "how in the world could ever you make that connection?"
"Well, Christ seems to be the paragon of good parenting, doesn't he? He's not saying if you're naughty, I'll give you a slap, nor even, as in the modern PC world, I'll withdraw your privileges, if you disobey me. He's saying, here's a moral way of looking at the world: if you think it's reasonable, take it on board and make it part of your own moral code. In other words, do the right thing because you believe it is the right thing, not because doing the wrong thing would risk incurring the wrath of someone else. He's teaching

us how to behave like adults, and in that sense, he's encouraging the development of the ego without undue censorship from the superego."
"Next thing you'll be telling me is that Christ was a Neo-Freudian psychoanalyst," said Jean-Paul.
"Well, maybe he was," said Matthew.

"Maybe you could try Epicurean philosophy," said Jean-Paul, "I think we both know that your Stoicism in the face of adversity was all just an act."
"You mean, indulge my emotions, for a change?"
"You can't live your life solely on an intellectual level, you know," said Jean-Paul, "you might as well be a cardboard cut-out."
"Is that all about 'emotional intelligence'?" asked Matthew. Jean-Paul sighed heavily, and then he tried to show Matthew what he was missing out on by conducting his existence solely in his head.
"Start to think with your guts," he said, "put all that ***angst*** to better use. I realise that neither fight nor flight is relevant in most twenty-first century encounters, but with a little practice you could learn to harness all that adrenalin and take on some new challenges. Who knows, you might actually enjoy the experience."

"So that's two dimensions dealt with: is there a third dimension?" asked Matthew. "You're actually in it now. Can you guess what it is?" said Jean-Paul, sounding vaguely like Rolf Harris. "I'll give you a clue: think of the multiple meanings of the German word, ***Geist.***" Matthew started to enumerate them:
"mind – is that the one?"
"Good guess, but not the crucial meaning."
"How about intellect – no we already have that dimension – then there's ghost: that sounds the closest to the English?"
"And another word for ghost is…", asked Jean-Paul.
"Spirit!" said Matthew, as the penny suddenly dropped. "Is there really such a thing as spiritual intelligence?"
"Of course there is: you can even do a spiritual IQ test, if you want. You'd probably come out as the ***investigative*** type: maybe you should have been a journalist.

But you see what I'm doing, don't you? I'm sowing the seeds of possible future challenges for you to consider once you have recovered. You're already well on your way to recovery. It may sound strange, but your break-down was the start of your recovery process. When your body and mind both say, 'I can't take any more!' they're making a conscious decision to change. Give them a month away from stress, some decent meals and a good night's sleep, and they'll be right as rain in no time at all. Forget the tranquillisers: they'll just arrest, or at best delay your recovery. Oh, and don't forget: no more cereals, and be especially wary of any foods with a high GI rating!"

"Now tell me," said Matthew, "how am I supposed to differentiate between treasure and fool's gold?" At this point, the voice of an ex-junky friend of Matthew's interrupted, reminiscing about his favourite weed, cannabis, "Moroccan Gold - that's good shit, man!"

"You see what I mean?" pointed out Jean-Paul, "A total contradiction in terms. But now, back to your studies, Matthew. So that you instinctively know what is worth keeping, I have arranged for you to study its very ***opposite***. Adopting the technique used by philosophers to define an item in terms of what it is not, you will begin a course of ***scatology*** – not, I hasten to add, to encourage you to take an unhealthy interest in coprophilia: I assume you had enough of that as an infant – and once you have a clear idea of what crap is, it should help you to separate the wheat from the chaff."

"Will I know ***kitsch*** when I see it?" asked Matthew.
"One man's kitsch is another man's souvenir with incalculable sentimental value," replied Jean-Paul, "but you will be able to apply your newly-acquired powers of discrimination to decide.
"And ***integrity***," said Matthew, "will I be able to detect that, say, in a politician?" Jean-Paul sighed,
"Oh yes, the so-called public servants, you mean? Just put it this way: if they've got their snouts in the trough, I wouldn't go offering them your pearls of wisdom!"

"Will I get any help from the psychiatrist?" asked Matthew.
"I wouldn't think so," said Jean-Paul, "They're so full of crap themselves, they're most unlikely to be able to help you!"

## Chapter thirty-two – the psychiatrist

***"The beauty of playing a psychiatrist is that it's a licence to be eccentric. It is one of the marvellous ironies that it's a job where you are helping the mentally unstable, yet it is the psychiatrists who often exhibit the most weirdness."***

**Stephen Fry, on playing this role in the American drama series, *Bones*.**

"We can't say for absolute certain, of course," said Suggs, "but the general consensus of the team is that you are what we nowadays call ***bipolar***. You may be more familiar with the term, manic-depressive. 'Suggs' was the nickname the inmates gave to Doctor Sugar, the psychiatrist at the hospital near York. It seemed quite appropriate that it was also the name of the lead singer with the band, Madness. In using Dr Sugar's nickname, the patients were effectively disempowering the professional. Had they addressed him by his correct title, ***Professor Sugar***, it would have been tantamount to saying, 'We acknowledge that in addressing you correctly we hereby grant you absolute power over us.'

Suggs continued,
"One question - just for the sake of clarification, you understand – do you hear voices?" Matthew went instinctively onto the defensive.
"If I say yes, you'll switch your diagnosis to schizophrenia, I presume?"
"Well, do you?" persisted the psychiatrist. Matthew was not about to go into detail about his conversations with Jean-Paul, for obvious reasons, so he opted for a more – shall we say – philosophical response.
"I take it you acknowledge that most folk with the basic remnants of morality have what is generally referred to as a conscience?"
"Go on," said the psychiatrist.
"I think the Church calls it 'that still small voice'. Though I am not a particularly religious person, I am happy to acknowledge that there may be a small region of the brain – let us call it the God-spot, for want of any better expression – that can intervene in our lives from time to time, when it thinks we are losing our way," explained Matthew.

"No malevolent whisperings? No persecuting demons? No one instructing you to do harm to yourself or others?" Suggs seemed almost disappointed. This did not appear to fit his style of convergent thinking. "Never mind: the distinction between the two diagnoses isn't that crucial: I'd place you as somewhere along that broad spectrum. I'm prescribing ***haloperidol*** – it works for both ends of the spectrum." Matthew remembered his G.P once prescribing a 'broad spectrum antibiotic'. When he asked for an explanation, Dr Martin was quite matter-of-fact. "I'm not quite sure what you have wrong with you, but this stuff is magic: it cures everything – you'll be better in no time."

"So how does the medication work?" Matthew asked the psychiatrist.
"That's for me to know and you to wonder at!" replied Dr Sugar, not entirely tongue-in-cheek. "Actually, we have made great strides forward in developing drugs to cure the mania; it's the depressive side we haven't had much luck with."
"Thanks a bunch!" said Matthew, "I much prefer the manic dimension."
"We need to slow everything down – those racing thoughts you're having, for example." Matthew was soon to discover what slowing everything down meant. The strong tranquiliser turned him into a virtual zombie, and within a month he had gained two stones in weight, seriously impacting on his already somewhat feeble heart. Other medication followed to counteract the side-effects of the first medication with yet another to alleviate the side-effects of the second or the combined interactions of medications one and two. The ***zopiclone*** was supposed to help him sleep: he managed no more than half-an-hour's sleep per night, despite huge doses of the drug.

"Are you sure you're a qualified analyst?" Matthew asked Suggs, the psychiatrist, "Not one of these dilettante ***oralists***, are you, telling me the reason I'm a control-freak is because I'm an only-child whom my mother overindulged? I suppose you're going to say that an only-child has no competition from siblings, and that is a very bad preparation for the cut-throat, dog-eat-dog world out there; that I'm a kind of 'id rules OK?' personality whose concept of ***ego*** was never properly developed and whose compliance with the norms of society as a consequence was largely down to the dominance of his ***superego***, or conscience, that his church upbringing had imposed on him?"

Suggs smiled, but said nothing. "Well, what are you going to tell me?" said Matthew, "that the reason why I'm such a defiant risk-taker; why I'm so disorganised and careless; why I'm so messy and obsessed by all kinds of crap is ultimately because I didn't get the right potty-training? Anal repulsive? Well, I'm proud of that aspect of my personality. Getting rid of all the crap from the past is the only way you can learn how to move on after traumatic events in your life. I'm not one for rehearsing all those past experiences in the hopes that the process will somehow exorcise the demons. I see so many folk trapped in the past. Some are still reliving the golden age of their childhood at the age of forty-four. Others cannot stop narrating their miserable life-experiences to everyone they meet, but yet seem blissfully unaware that nobody wants to hear that stuff, often for the second or third time."

"We want you to stop indulging these delusory ideas," said Suggs, "otherwise you're going to lose your grip on reality entirely."

"Who's to say they're delusory?" retorted Matthew, angry that the ***thought-police*** were interfering in his own peculiar way of looking at the world. Even the meaning of the word 'dream' was ambiguous. Was it a joyful experience, like a reverie, or did it trip over into delirium? Jean-Paul came to his defence, suggesting Matthew tell the psychiatrist to read Aldous Huxley's ***Doors of Perception***. "Just because you shut out ninety-five per cent of what's out there doesn't negate its existence," said Matthew. "Having expanded my mind to accommodate perhaps a 180 degree experience, as compared to your 18 degree view of the world, it is my contention that I can lead a much fuller life as a result. Okay, maybe you occasionally allow as much as a 50 degree angle into your eyes, about as much as the average camera lens, but when your eyes are capable of seeing a much wider angle, and at a far higher resolution than any camera, why do you allow your brain to filter it all out?"

Suggs agreed to read the book, but returned to his agenda,
"And are you still hearing the voices?" Matthew thought this trick question had deliberately been smuggled in at the last minute. We know that he had intentionally avoided telling the psychiatrist about the voices to steer clear of being categorised as a schizophrenic. And had he added his tendency towards catatonic fits and violent outbursts, the diagnosis would most likely have been confirmed.
"I never said I heard voices," said Matthew, "but since one in ten of ***normal*** people admit to hearing voices, what's the great crime here, Mr Thought-policeman?" Suggs momentarily adopted an empathetic mode,
"You do realise that the voices usually talk people into harming either themselves or others, don't you?" said the psychiatrist.

"It depends on how you handle your anger," said Matthew. "I can take it out on a drum-kit or a guitar. Some folk channel it into painting, others into drama or writing. I am convinced that the voices are just an example of healthy debate. You probably call it 'internal conflict'. Once you accept the world to be a set of finely balanced paradoxes, you can live with the contradictions. The voices can be generated through early religious indoctrination. People of my generation still have a conscience, so if we had become politicians, we would have resisted the temptation to milk the system to feather our own nests, because we would have still had a moral compass."
"Oh, yes," said the psychiatrist, "and pigs might fly!" Matthew sighed, mixing his metaphors somewhat,
"Not whilst they have the opportunity to keep their snouts in the trough, no. You're so cynical, you doctors, don't you allow for altruistic idealists at all in your world?" Suggs smiled.
"That's rich, coming from you, the arch-cynic!" he mused.

"So who are these non-religious voices of yours?" asked Suggs.

"Some are just like mischievous children," said Matthew. "The little devils come to call when you've been taking everything far too seriously for too long. So long as you don't let it get out of hand, it's usually harmless fun, and they help you to gain a sense of perspective on life." Picking up on Matthew's words, the psychiatrist decided to push it further,
"And has it ever got ***out of hand***?" Matthew paused to evaluate whether to spill the beans or keep quiet about the game of 'truth or dare'. Not wishing to provide ammunition for the doctor's case, he elected for the latter course of action, moving on to the origins of other voices.
"It's all about authority figures," Matthew said, "in a way, they're all variations on the same theme. I suppose they're like the ***superego*** in your world."

"How was the relationship with your father?" asked the psychiatrist.
"Quite good, I suppose," said Matthew, "though he wasn't what you would usually regard as an authority figure. I do remember him always standing up for me in school and other parents were impressed by his courage in taking on some quite formidable teachers. He tried desperately to inculcate in me a respect for authority, but I was having none of it. I was prepared to acknowledge a modicum of respect simply because of the ***position*** an individual held, but that didn't stop me regarding the ***person*** as beneath contempt."

Becoming a teacher helped Matthew to dispel the aura he had attributed to the profession as a kid. He still experienced inexplicable paranoia in connection with all professions in the sphere of jurisprudence. When it comes to the Day of Judgement, we will all be our own worst critics. The voice of the judge was the epitome of this self-destructive streak in him. He could only make it go away by projecting judgemental comments onto others. The voice of reason was always conspicuous by his or her absence from the cacophonous choir of whisperers. Perhaps Jean-Paul was unique in that respect: he was the only one of Matthew's voices that represented the voice of reason.

## Chapter thirty-three – the thinker

Now, Matthew was well aware that, in Suggs' words, nine times out of ten, hearing voices can lead you to follow their malevolent suggestions (e.g. The Yorkshire Ripper), yet this particular voice seemed trustworthy. Any good counsellor worth his or her salt will offer a variety of choices so that the clients effectively decide for themselves on a course of action. One advantage for the counsellors is that they cannot subsequently be blamed for the suggested course of action and the clients must take ownership of their decisions. Jean-Paul was such a counsellor. He showed Matthew how to find his own way out of the wilderness.

It was Jean-Paul who explained how to start making sense of language through putting like with like and rejecting misleading concepts.
"Take swearing, for example," said Jean-Paul, "Do you think it is wrong to swear, Matthew?"
"I hadn't really given it much thought," replied Matthew, "I don't actually swear much, myself, though it's not because I find it morally repugnant; it just seems such a waste of words when there are several hundred thousand more appropriate ones out there at our disposal."

Matthew found it easy to swear in foreign languages: the words themselves clearly did not have the same impact on him as swear-words in his own language. Jean-Paul chose his next argument carefully for maximum effect.
"Take ***fucking hell*** or ***holy shit***, for example," he proposed.
"Spirits are not supposed to talk like that!" exclaimed Matthew, somewhat shocked, "I thought spirit guides would keep well away from such expressions."
"This is a philosophical debate, where the expressions I have just used have been carefully selected to illustrate a point,"
"Which is...?" asked Matthew. Jean-Paul went on to show Matthew how people's brains have been polluted by a random mix of expletives from unconnected sources. "You have scatological vocabulary combined with the religious or sexual expressions. Not only that, you link a positive with a negative connotation – how can your brain possibly make sense of such an oxymoron? If you are going to ***toilet mouth*** – to use the vernacular of the citizens' broadcast radio – keep it to that category alone. Religious swear-words have lost their original meaning: bloody is short for ***By Our Lady*** but now seems to have been relegated to a class B profanity. And if you ask me, the proliferation of the f-word has totally disassociated it from its original connection with sex."

During psychoanalysis, Matthew kept coming back to texts he had studied, relating to the process of reflection. It did rather seem, however, that he took the notion of 'thinking about thinking' to extremes. He was not content to get his head round ***metacognition***, the technical term for this process, but progressed one step further into ***hypermetacognition***, a term he himself coined for the process he had invented. Analysis can sometimes be a really destructive process, but, when everything has been cut back to just the bare essentials, with all the unnecessary elaboration stripped away, you can be left with the basic necessities for a very good life.

Throughout the period when his dreams, reveries and nightmares were trying to accommodate a wealth of intellectual argument, at the same time as he was on an emotional roller-coaster, the Beatles song, ***All you need is Love***, kept on playing in the background, in his head, and deep inside he knew that ***love*** would ultimately be his salvation. Whilst he sensed his intellectual psyche disintegrating at the one extreme, he could feel the message coming through loud and clear that his emotional self would prevail as a compensatory force, at the other extreme.

Alice had warned Matthew not to return to the super-analytical process of self-reflection that practically destroyed him last time, yet Jean-Paul had seemed to be actually encouraging him to deconstruct everything. That analysis of profanities had been a start.
"Come on, Jean-Paul," said Matthew, "I'm doing the psychoanalysis all on my own!" "That's the whole point," said Jean-Paul, "it's rather like hypnosis, you know, you've tried that, haven't you? Don't you remember how it was really all about ***self-hypnosis***? Nothing to do with the hypnotist having some Svengali hold or Mesmeric spell over someone – more about how prepared the subject was to go along with the whole charade. Do you remember doing the ***will she? / won't she?*** test on your subjects? If she was up for it, she tended to move back as you approached her, but if she stood her ground, it meant she was unlikely to be a good subject, because she was likely to be more resistant. You gradually realised that you could induce a form of self-hypnosis upon yourself. I remember laughing out loud when you refused to let anyone hypnotise ***you*** – were you afraid of losing control, perhaps?

Anyway, as I was saying before I got distracted and went off at a tangent; analysis is like hypnosis because it's really a do-it-yourself therapy. Do you really need a shrink to present you with the set of stimulus words? Just try it: even a random set of words will help to get you focussed." Matthew began with some innocuous-looking words, just to see where the word-association game led him. Whenever Matthew reached 'the end-of-the-line', Jean-Paul would suggest he go back a word, and start a new train of connections. Bizarre links would be noted, and predictable associations ignored. In much the same way as he had encouraged Matthew to separate out the swear-words into scatological, sexual and religious categories, Jean-Paul taught him the error of confused thinking, "Remember how the Nazis tried to control thinking with perverse logic such as ***Arbeit macht frei***,[19] the slogan placed above the entrance to the concentration camp. Beware the latter-day spin-doctors who invent terms such as ***collateral damage*** and ***quantitative easing***: it's all designed to keep you in the dark and not question the real meaning of the expressions. Eventually, you'll start bandying these phrases about like everyone else, even though you'll have become oblivious to the normalisation in society they have engendered in that process. I can remember you yourself getting onto the band-wagon with your '***paradigm-shift***,' long before you'd grasped its meaning, just to impress the panel by pretending to show you were speaking their language."

"The danger is that our whole society gets fucked up through trying to communicate in code."
"Mind your language!" cautioned Matthew.
"That's unfortunately the way it is. Mental illness is on the rise, partly because people just don't have the vocabulary with which to communicate. Researchers in America actually found it therapeutic to teach German to their mental patients. Must have had something to do with the basic simplicity of the language. Take ***epistemology***, for example, any idea what it is?"
"My knowledge of Greek doesn't stretch that far," said Matthew.
"Perhaps you'd find its German equivalent, ***Erkenntnistheorie,*** easier to decipher, even though it's not your native tongue. Quite obvious, when you understand the component words: ***theory of knowledge***. The problem with English is that it comes from so many other languages, and, not knowing the original meanings of the root-words, no two people can guarantee they are talking about the same thing when they use an expression."

Matthew found this happened with basic concepts and hackneyed phrases, too. The expression, ***place of safety***, for example, would be synonymous with a safe haven or sanctuary to a psychiatric patient needing to escape from his trauma, whilst, for the 'professionals' it might more closely resemble a prison-cell or a locked ward. This mismatch between the idea the controllers had in their minds and the idea 'users' had, led to great misunderstandings at meetings that had been designed to give patients more say in their treatment.

---

[19] Work makes you free

## Chapter thirty-four – the insider

Matthew spent much of his life as an outsider and consequently he empathised very much with those living on the margins of society. There is nothing worse than feeling excluded. It might be that you are rejected by the clique for some inexplicable reason. Matthew always believed this to be true. That is, until he was obliged to spend time in a psychiatric institution.

Matthew went straight from playing the role of the outsider, looking in, to the insider, looking out, cutting out the middle-man altogether. Deciding that discretion was the better part of valour, Matthew elected to have 'voluntary' psychiatric treatment, because he was well aware of the consequences of being sectioned. Though, at the time, he did not have sufficient 'insight' to appreciate the need for his incarceration, he had to acknowledge that if he remained in this state of hypomania much longer, he would probably die of a heart attack. He willingly took the narcosis-inducing drugs, because he really appreciated the couple of hours sleep per night they provided, but he took the other sedatives and tranquillisers with extreme reluctance, failing to see how zombie status could help the individual, however much more manageable he became for the staff as a patient, under the 'chemical cosh'.

In the hospital, as Matthew was quickly to learn, there were three ***regimes*** operating simultaneously. He encountered the first of these immediately on arrival. It felt like he imagined army life to be. At six o'clock in the morning, he was ordered to report to the wash-rooms where he was handed the necessary towel and soap. After a quick shower, shave and a passing acquaintance with his toothbrush, he and his fellow lab-rats were urged to dress appropriately and then report to the refectory for breakfast. It was going to be a very long day ahead, he rightly assumed. He did not like this situation at all, and devised a number of coping strategies.

One of these was an idea inspired by Oskar, the main character in ***The Tin Drum*** by Gunther Grass, who refused to speak. Matthew realised that in his present unguarded manic phase, he might unwittingly incriminate himself, prolonging the incarceration, or hastening the administration of even more powerful and toxic drugs than he was on already. He would feign muteness, he decided. Armed with a small note book, he would write down questions for the psychiatric team. Had he posed the same questions verbally, they would have reminded him that it was their job to ask the questions, his simply to respond truthfully. The notebook somewhat reversed the two roles and he was able to glean quite a large amount of information about his condition.

Soon he was moved to a separate wing of the Victorian hospital. He adored the architecture and was delighted by the sun shining in through the stained glass windows. The policy seemed to be to pair him up with other inmates for a couple of days at a time; not long enough for him to work out any kind of escape strategy by conspiring with a potential would-be escapee. On this occasion, the ***regime*** was one of ***laissez-faire***. No one bothered what time you got up or went to bed; the only thing they checked on was that you took your medication and ate your food. The boredom was relieved by frequent walks up and down the corridors to make endless cups of coffee. No attempt had been made to segregate the sexes which seemed more humanising for the men, but rather intimidating for some of the women. The tedium was sporadically interrupted by impromptu entertainment. One day, one poor fellow felt an uncontrollable desire to rescue some plastic flowers from the bin, but then proceeded to remove his pyjamas in full view of the assembled company. Another day, a trainee female psychiatrist appeared on the ward having forgotten to display her I.D. card. Since she was not wearing the trappings of her profession, two psychiatric nurses, who had not been informed of her arrival, promptly seized her arms to take her to one of the other wings. (If a patient strayed from their allocated wing, they were taken back there by the staff).
"Take your hands off me!" she exclaimed with great indignation, "Don't you realise who I am? – I'm the eminent psychiatrist, Doctor Emilia Schwarzkopf!" One of the nurses smiled, knowingly.
"That's what they all say, dear, I wasn't born yesterday, you know." Eventually, all the hullabaloo attracted the attention of a passing psychiatrist, and, after reassurances from him that she was indeed a genuine doctor, she was released.

Paranoia was palpable on the ward. Doctors did not like patients undermining their efforts by giving each other alternative diagnoses and prognoses. There was, therefore, always the suspicion that one of the patients might be a plant, trying to get information, and when Gilbert arrived, dressed - in the estimation of the rest of them just like another psychiatrist - in his suit and tie, everyone was on their guard. Matthew was the first to speak with him. You can generally spot a fraud. Certainly, most newly-admitted patients are still high; their faces virtually glow and were they not mad, you would probably say they emanated charisma, a halo almost. Gilbert's ***holy shine*** was still in evidence and it transpired that he was actually the son of a psychiatrist.

For obvious reasons, psychiatrists themselves rarely feel free to practice what they preach by submitting themselves for treatment whenever they go over the edge. If they do actually get sectioned, there are special hospitals where they can be given treatment. After all, it just would not do for them to mix with the ***hoi polloi*** , and just think how it would undermine the confidence of one of the other patients if he or she were to meet their former shrink in the loony-bin. History suggests most of them just continue their psychiatric practice, relying on their unquestionable status to protect them from removal from power.

"Lose the tie!" Matthew suggested, in a rather unsubtle way, encouraging Gilbert to adopt the more conventional uniform of jeans and a sweatshirt. As he observed the inmates gradually coming down from their highs, or, alternatively, approaching the hyper stage after passing through the less bizarre hypomania, his thoughts strayed to an analogy with the video camera.
"The cameraman sits aboard a vehicle equipped with suitable hydraulics so that he can ***elevate*** to achieve a superior view of a scene, or ***depress*** to return to ground level. This effectively mirrors the two extremes of the bipolar condition."
"Every analogy breaks down, eventually," Gilbert protested, but Matthew asked him to bear with him for a moment.
"The camera," said Matthew, "can pan left or right, and so can the brain; it can zoom in up close and personal, very much in-your-face, focussing solely on the detail, or it can zoom out to see the whole picture. It can also tilt up or down, and even roll over, if you wish. Don't you think the human being behaves similarly?"
"You need to give more examples," said Gilbert.
"A simple example is the way we talk about looking up to, or admiring people, and looking down on people or despising them. In films, the camera angle indicates who is the victim down in the gutter, and who is the powerful person up on an imaginary pedestal."

A further diversion was caused when a clearly distressed lady came in shouting, "Give me the electricity! I need the electricity." It emerged that this was the third experimental ***regime*** in the hospital. Matthew found the whole notion that electro-convulsive therapy was still being administered in the year 2000 barbaric; he found it even more bizarre that patients were clamouring for it. In the early days, it was administered without anaesthetic, with something stuffed in your mouth to stop you biting your tongue. It was the apparent randomness of treatment in this hospital that puzzled Matthew. Was there any reason why he had been spared this form of torture? Talking to his friends, for now within this microcosm the other inmates were all he had to socialise with, Matthew discovered which responses guaranteed extensions to your sentence and which responses offered the best chance of ***parole***.
"If it looks like a prison and feels like a prison, then it is a prison," said Matthew, after, unusually, all the doors had been locked one night.
"Word is going round, there's a killer in our midst," whispered Gilbert, and sure enough, when the doors were unlocked the following morning, Dave was no longer with them. "He must have been the killer," said Gilbert.

"He seemed a perfectly okay kind of guy to me," said Matthew, who was now temporarily without a room-mate.

So far, we have only had brief glimpses into Matthew's alternative reality. Just as 'normality' is defined as that which the majority consider normal, so it is with reality when society reaches a general consensus about what is real. Take the Soviet Union under communism, for example. As we know, Matthew's drug, ***haloperidol,*** which was once used to tranquilise horses, (as well as to dissuade parrots from plucking out their feathers) came to be used in the West to treat schizophrenia and manic depression. In Russia, the same drug was used to attempt to 'cure' dissidents of capitalist thinking. We can assume that the thinking of true communists was: how could anyone possibly want any other kind of utopia? What could be wrong with seeking equality for all? Anyone who wanted more than his neighbour clearly needed such deviant thoughts expunged from his psyche.

Contrasting the capitalist and communist excuses for administering this drug, one might suspect that, like most medication, it was not designed as a therapeutic treatment for the psychotic individual, but rather as a means of control: certainly, its widespread use in institutions is legendary – how much easier it is to manage the sick when they are heavily sedated and hence not as likely to cause a nuisance. If we think there is any real freedom of expression in ***our*** country, we need to think again. As the definition of what is normal becomes ever more narrowly defined, we will see the virtual extinction of the eccentric personality, whose only crime might be to want an alternative lifestyle which would not unduly impinge on the lives of his fellow men.

Ironically, the ambit of reality has gone in the opposite direction: the definition has broadened. Imagine twenty-first century man transported back in time just fifty years. Imagine he took with him all the paraphernalia that people nowadays deem indispensable: very quickly, he would probably be assigned to a loony-bin for talking to himself in the street (using a mobile phone). Imagine if he enumerated all those imaginary friends he had on facebook: might the psychiatrists of the day not - with some justification - have deemed him insane and living in a fantasy world? Had he mentioned ***Second Life*** where his avatar could function every bit as well, if not better than his mundane normal persona, they would have had him sectioned immediately. Yet now, fifty years later, such behaviour has become normalised. Just like the eccentrics, the traditionalists will be swept aside by technological advances, rendering their normality abnormal: normality is all about the view of the majority. (The next target group for the psychiatrists and the pharmaceutical giants they support has already been decided: the obese).

"You're coming up before the parole board tomorrow," observed Gilbert, "Do you want to rehearse your lines?"
"Great idea!" said Matthew.
"You sound too optimistic already," remarked Gilbert, "Tone it down a bit. Now, here's the crucial question, how do you ***feel***?"
"I feel fine," said Matthew, expressing what he felt to be the truth.
"Wrong answer!" retorted Gilbert. You should have said something like, 'it's getting a bit better'. Obviously, there's no point in going to the opposite extreme and saying 'awful', but showing that you realise you still have a long way to go on the road to recovery – no, wait a minute, on second thoughts, don't ever mention the "r" word, they don't like that. It implies that you will be dispensing with their services and that would put them all out of work."

The hospital was - perhaps surprisingly - tolerant, in Matthew's estimation, of alternative therapies. On the programme for the day appeared yoga, reflexology, and aromatherapy in addition to art and pottery, badminton and relaxation CD's. After getting initial two-hour passes followed by overnight passes to stay with his family, Matthew gradually re-accustomed himself to the speed of the rat-race that was normality. He decided to brave the consequences of going ***cold turkey*** on his medication as soon as he was out of the sight of those supervising compliance. Anita was at once encouraging, yet fearful, as she had no experience of what to expect. The medication is generally administered over a six month period. Anyone attempting to come off it is warned of the dangers of so doing, and many quickly resume their poison once the doctor catches them out, pointing out the error of their ways. They are forced to recant and admit that the doctor knew best after all. Matthew stopped after six weeks.

It went surprisingly well, all things considered. Matthew undertook to paint the garden fencing panels as a way of keeping his mind off the withdrawal symptoms. Normally, in his decorating days, he could have polished the whole job off in a couple of days, but physically, all he could manage was one panel per day and there were thirty of them.
"All done!" he chirped triumphantly, exactly one month after leaving hospital. He no longer experienced the nausea, the tremors, the anxiety, the collywobbles, screaming habdabs or heebie-jeebies that preyed on him during his period of detoxification. He continued to collect repeat prescriptions for the following three months, but never took them to the chemist to be filled. As a consequence, his body and soul started to heal themselves.

At the follow-up appointment with Dr Scott, his psychiatrist, six months later, Matthew was deemed to have recovered sufficiently to be able to resume his teaching duties. Again, at this meeting, as he had in the hospital, he subtly exchanged roles with the doctor, taking an interest in the unsuspecting gentleman's family and hobbies. After being granted the somewhat rare opportunity to offload some of his own personal issues, the psychiatrist quickly realised that Matthew was now as sane as the next man and refrained from his usual routine of prescribing more long-term medications such as lithium injections.

"How are your stocks and shares doing, at the moment?" asked Matthew, pushing his luck somewhat, he felt. In an unguarded moment, Dr Scott instinctively responded to the request,
"Upjohn are doing very well; Pfizer and Eli Lilly are performing as anticipated." This information confirmed what Matthew had long suspected: a cosy relationship between the psychiatrists and the pharmaceutical companies. Matthew tried another exploratory question:
"Is it true that British psychiatrists have to give diagnoses laid down by their American counterparts, even though the Brits no longer believe certain psychiatric conditions exist?"

Dr Scott was surprised that Matthew had heard of such agreements,
"I take it you're referring to bipolar? It's true we don't tend to diagnose it so readily in the UK as the Americans do in their home country, but why do you ask?" Matthew, as we know, had been diagnosed bipolar and therefore, quite reasonably, wanted to know what might now happen to his 'label'.
"I felt comfortable with bipolar – it had almost become fashionable amongst the celebrities, but now I would seem to be in limbo." Dr Scott tried to reassure him,
"I know how important it is to be given a diagnosis, whether of a psychiatric or a physical illness. I suggest we reclassify you as a schizophrenic, or borderline personality disorder, if you like – it's only a label after all." Matthew frowned,
"So you won't let me off with just being an ***eccentric***, then?"

Matthew did not like answering questions, but, as a teacher, he had mostly been in the role of interrogator. Now he was about to find the roles reversed.

## Chapter thirty-five – the Inquisitor

Despite knowing the inherent dangers of thinking about thinking, as Robbie Williams calls ***metacognition***, Matthew allowed himself the indulgence of his own version of self-psychoanalysis, adopting quick-fire sequences where the stimulus word would yield the occasional bizarre connection. He took a mental note of these, but continued with the game until he ran out of ideas. At this point, he would train his mind to go back to the last connection and then follow a new path of connections. It was during this Aristotelian categorisation that he stumbled on the six question words. What were the relative merits of these, he wondered?

"What's the best way of getting to the bottom of my muddled way of thinking and start to put it back in order?" asked Matthew. Jean-Paul read out the following poem:

**I keep six honest serving-men**
**(They taught me all I knew);**
**Their names are What and Why and When**
**And How and Where and Who.**

**Rudyard Kipling – the Elephant's Child.**

"Basically, question-words are really the quintessence of what communication is all about," said Jean-Paul. Matthew had been striving to analyse meaning to the nth degree. "You are well aware of the destructive power of analysis," continued Jean-Paul. "Do you remember how, as a child - like all young boys – you dismantled your toys to see how they worked?" Matthew remembered very well:
"But I had always followed it up with reconstruction. I liked the satisfaction of fixing broken things." Jean-Paul was impressed,
"Perhaps later, you will be able to apply that same determination in your endeavours to mend broken people."

"You must start by prioritising your own personal choices," said Jean-Paul. Not surprisingly, the question, ***how***, emerged as Matthew's favourite question word. After all, this chimed in with his practical bent. From an educational point of view, he had observed teaching methodologies come and go, even return, so he could see where the current preoccupation with ***skills*** fitted in.
"My own education centred almost exclusively on the ***what,***." said Matthew.
"Facts are a virtual irrelevance nowadays: You can search for all that kind of stuff on the internet," said Jean-Paul.

"But don't we need a combination of knowledge, skills and ***understanding***?" asked Matthew.
"Yes, of course, there's that tricky question word, ***why***, as well, isn't there?" said Jean-Paul.

"Who are you?" demanded Jean-Paul, the spirit guide, as Matthew embarked upon an intensive period of self-analysis, triggered after a particularly ***florid*** manic episode.
"I'm a Head of Department in a University," he replied.
"That's not what I asked!" responded Jean-Paul.
"What do you mean?" Matthew enquired.
"I didn't ask you ***what*** you do; I asked you ***who*** you are! It's not about status or titles."
"I really don't get what you mean," Matthew protested.
"Until you can say honestly, and with all humility, ***'this is me – warts and all'*** – you won't ever be able to answer that question," explained Jean-Paul.

This gave Matthew an awful lot of things to mull over in both the waking and sleeping hours ahead, but Jean-Paul had counselled him to be very wary about the information he divulged to psychiatrists, so he decided to keep it to himself, only committing coded messages to his note-book for future reference in case his memory failed him.

## Chapter thirty-six – the codifier

Mathematicians would appear to inhabit a twilight world on the edge of reality, frequently relying on dreams to solve perplexing problems. Kekulé is alleged to have discovered the formula for benzene after dreaming of a snake with its tail in its mouth, for instance. Matthew found that 'sleeping on it' occasionally worked in solving crossword puzzles whose enigmatic clues totally flummoxed him the day before. Almost immediately on picking up the paper the next day, he had the answers.

At the time of decimalisation of sterling, in the early nineteen-seventies, when Matthew had been a student, he had wondered how long it would be before time itself was decimalised. He experimented with units of time, but there was no way a week could be conveniently split up into ten segments. Of course, before Julius and Augustus came along, folk had managed perfectly well with ten months (viz ***Dec***ember), but Matthew kept dwelling on the French/German notion of huit jours / acht Tage, and wondered if that was where the Beatles had got their idea for the song, ***Eight Days a Week***, having spent some considerable time in Hamburg, as they had. He promptly devised his own eight-day week, each day conveniently made up of twenty-one hours so that eight of his days were exactly the same as seven normal days. He invented names for these days: solidas, lunidas, maridas, demidas, gravidas, venidas, saturdas, and jovidas.

There was little difference at the start of the week - Matthew would stay up for fourteen hours and sleep for seven – but by the end of his week, most of his 'day' was during the night, and vice versa. As a student, he could implement this regime, as he only had lectures on the first three days. Apart from a degree of disorientation when he started the scheme, he found it most productive, allowing, as it did, one more day of study than his colleagues had. Maybe it paved the way for the time when, ten years later, his Master's dissertation had to be completed over a ten day period; for, luckily, this burst of activity coincided with one of his more manic phases, when he was super-alert.

Just as Matthew had discovered that an eight-day week composed of 21-hour days was the same as a normal seven-day week (i.e.168 hours), so he also found that you could theoretically have a six day week comprising 28-hour days, but after who'sday, when'sday, where'sday, whyday and whataday, he decided he had had a very questionable week already, and gave up on 'howday' altogether!

He loved the number nine, that spiritual number that always resolves to nine, numerologically speaking, no matter how many multiples of it you consider:

18=9; 27=9; 36=9; 45=9; 54=9; 63=9; 72=9; 81=9; etc

This fascination with numbers escalated with his illness. Prior to the breakdown, his mathematical abilities were minimal. He now took to studying packs of playing cards and decided to challenge his friends to a game. Again, he had always been useless at cards, losing virtually every game he played, regardless of the hand he was dealt; but now he was beating the others hands down. His brain seemed to be more alert and, moreover, he did not even have to try. In addition, the individual playing cards took on a more sinister connotation as their symbolic values became clear to him. Friends and relatives were identified according to their influence.[20] Someone with financial potential might be the king of diamonds, for example; hearts obviously represented love, but then there was that most inauspicious of cards, the nine of spades, a card to be tactfully avoided. He felt in some way that the cards were helping him to bring order into his brain. Just the simple routine of laying out the cards every day in the hospital seemed to help.

Just as mathematicians use a shorthand, Matthew devised his own set of symbols[21] to identify the degrees of integrity of his colleagues. As his boss had pointed out, this would normally have been deemed a matter for disciplinary action, had he been in his right mind at the time. The millennium may not have triggered the anticipated meltdown of the World Wide Web, as in Y2K, but it did seem to herald a surge in the number of individuals admitted to psychiatric institutions. Matthew put it down to folk with delusions of grandeur adopting Messianic roles in anticipation of the end of the world.

Matthew, in his state of hypomania, was perplexed. His right brain, which had temporarily taken over the management of his affairs, was dictating the need for candour, yet whatever remained of his left brain urged caution. Consequently, his paranoia grew and he genuinely felt that he could no longer trust a single individual in his ambit of contacts and relations. "Trust only Alice," it urged, though Alice herself might have deemed this unwise advice, because in Matthew's present state she would have done whatever she felt necessary to ensure his safety, even if this meant breaking a confidence, which might, at least in theory, lead to him being sectioned.

In the hospital, writing in encrypted form enabled Matthew to keep a record without – as he saw it – incriminating himself. This was powerful stuff, after all; he didn't want it to be consigned to oblivion, because the medical profession thought the waters of Lethe were the best way of ensuring his

---

[20] See Appendix (i)
[21] See Appendix (ii)

recovery. Now there's an interesting way of looking at mental health: they want to put you back to how you used to be – "nice to see you're returning to your old self, at last," they would say, whilst deep inside Matthew knew that going back was the last thing he needed to do. He needed to move forward, and this could only come through re-inventing himself. He could understand the point of the narcotics – he needed to sleep, just to survive; and tranquilisers – yes, he could see the need to reduce his anxiety levels, though not to the extent of sedating him into a comatose state. He did not wish to be ***restored*** to his former self at all. Strange word ***psychosis***. Literally, it means giving life to [Greek psukhosis]. Might account for the animism, he thought.

**Chapter thirty-seven – the animist**

Assuming the reader is prepared to suspend disbelief, Matthew will now lead you gently by the hand, if not by the nose, into the somewhat bewildering, yet fascinating fantasy world of ***animism***, where inanimate objects take on the symbolic features of living creatures.

Waking up in his hospital bed, Matthew had suddenly felt hypersensitive and deeply emotional.
"Probably something to do with my previous existence, permeated as it was with bouts of insensitivity to my fellow human beings. I was brought up to keep a 'stiff upper lip' and I took a pride in not registering any pain or exhibiting any emotion throughout my life," he said to Dave, his room-mate. Dave, like any other sentient being, needed clarification,
"Are you suggesting a process of compensation?" Matthew suddenly felt an incredible urge to hug this relative stranger. What was that all about? There certainly was no physical attraction there. He had experienced similar inclinations at work, prior to his hospitalisation, but it applied equally to males and females, sometimes even plants. Colleagues had reported having felt his arm around them. Though this invasion of body space was generally discouraged at work, there were a number of colleagues who routinely used touch, rather like Prime Ministers do, to assert their control over their minions, but Matthew had always been so distant; not a touch-feely kind of person at all: it was the fact that this behaviour was unusual in his case that got folk worrying he might start making advances of a more sexual nature towards them.

What Matthew found even more bizarre, however, was his sudden attachment to inanimate objects, rather like his friend in the hospital who rescued the plastic flowers. Luckily for Matthew, this was not accompanied by a desire to strip off. Instead, he carefully picked out his toothbrush and razor, imagining that they had somehow acquired an element of life, like crudely arranged fresh fruit set out for a still life painting. Other household items had similarly acquired great significance: a broken lamp, an oil-burner, and an old Morphy- Richards iron were identified as crucial travelling companions when he took the train south. Anyone opening his case would have been puzzled by the abundance of useless items as compared to the bare minimum of essentials, such as a wash bag and a change of underwear.

Dave was finding this attachment to inanimate objects bewildering, to say the least. "How can you relate to a broken lamp, for example," he asked. "
Surely ***you*** must have developed a sentimental attachment to one of your possessions at some point in your life," suggested Matthew, "a cuddly toy, a

gift from someone now deceased, or a keepsake from a former girlfriend, perhaps?"
"I see what you mean," said Dave, suddenly understanding where Matthew was coming from, "like me being in love with my sports-car?"
"Now you're mixing it up with your ***alter ego*** and consumerism. You need to abandon the notion of material possessions. The items I'm thinking of evoke deep emotions within me: there's no logical reason for it – maybe it's just my emotions desperately seeking something to focus on and the inanimate objects simply represent a symbol for something entirely different." Dave thought about what he had once heard about phobias.
"You know arachnophobia," he began, "they reckon most people pick it up when something traumatic happens in their lives. The phobia's there to mask the real fear, which is of something much worse."

Matthew tried to recall all that Freudian psychoanalysis that he had once studied. It did not come flashing back as he had hoped. Instead, he recalled notions of projection: how you can so easily see a fault in your colleague, because it is one you yourself are guilty of.
"If you can project onto people, perhaps you can equally well project onto things," he stated. "These broken items may symbolise the externalisation of my love for the people they represent – they're all items inextricably linked to the members of my immediate family."

What was the symbolic significance of the fact that each of these items was broken? Did it represent the damage he had caused to the people they represented by his overbearing, censorial authoritarianism? He was about to find out.

## Chapter thirty-eight – the judge

**Judge not, lest ye yourselves be judged**
**Matthew, 7**

Mark wondered whether he might have inherited certain aspects of his father's bipolar condition and he reflected on some of the behaviour patterns he had observed in his father as he grew up. The diagnosis had not come until his father was already into his fifties, when Mark himself was in his late twenties. The family had occasionally been somewhat dysfunctional, though, in the circumstances, Mark did not feel he had much to complain about. He had long since forgiven, though not forgotten, his father's violent outbursts, preferring to remember instead– with hindsight - one amusing incident.

"You mustn't cry, Mark," his mother had said, "nobody got hurt." The entire contents of a plate of fish and chips, launched, as usual, in a rather clumsy fashion by Matthew, had narrowly missed his mother's face. Mark, the child, had exclaimed,
"I'm very hungry, and now I'm not going to get any dinner!"
"Don't get upset, Mark," said Matthew, in a contrite attempt to reassure his son. "I'll cook us all something else."

Mark recalled his father seemingly getting wound up by something his mother had said, and then suddenly exploding for no apparent reason. On one occasion, Matthew had ripped the banister right away from the staircase. Of course, he had immediately apologised and set about repairing the damage.
"Dad's been having a hard time at work, Mark," said his mother. "I think it's a case of 'kick-the-dog' syndrome." Mark was outraged to think that people could talk about mistreating animals in such a casual way. Looking back, as an adult, he realised that maybe his father had been in the wrong job, or, alternatively, should have been referred to a psychiatrist earlier. It seemed to him that the family had all conspired - his mother, his sister and himself - to disguise his father's condition by virtually normalising his behaviour.

Matthew's daughter, Kate, had herself enjoyed – if that is the right word for it – the benefit of several months undergoing psychotherapy. As a consequence, she took on board many of the theories as well as some of the tricks of the trade. She vowed that one day she would put all of these skills to practical use. One of the pieces of advice had been to 'avoid the negative'. By this she understood that the way to liberate herself was to break free from the stiflingly judgemental figures in her life. As she was growing up, there was the inevitable sibling rivalry and she had the impression that she could never match up to the achievements of her elder brother, at least not in her father's eyes. She imagined her brother would probably just copy the way his father would orchestrate, often in the full public gaze, the calculated put-down of some ***poor defenceless female,*** though she vowed no such label would ever apply to her.

Her father was the typical male chauvinist pig, in many ways. She felt sorry for her mother who seemed to be the only person pulling her weight in the household, doing all the chores, whilst her father had the gall to lie full-length on the sofa, watching TV. And yet, he was the one always meting out the criticism. She sometimes felt like voicing her opinion on the subject. In her head she would be saying,
"What gives you the right to complain about other people's failings, when you can't succeed at your own job?" Secretly, she wished he had offered her – and her brother, for that matter - a better role-model of what an ideal ***man*** would be: she would have liked nothing better than to have had a proper father to indulge her, like the fathers her friends seemed to have.

Her brother, Mark, seemed to be the blue-eyed boy for his father; for he could do nothing wrong. Mark picked up the same belittling attitude to women that his father had. The pair of them were a couple of misogynists. When her mother tactfully suggested to Matthew from time to time to praise or flatter his daughter, he seemed at a loss to understand how to do that, and ended up making what his own father probably would have called a 'back-handed compliment'. His pusillanimity was boundless. Anyway, what value was there in a compliment that had to be prompted? She felt unloved. With a father who abuses through neglect, what prospect does a girl have of finding a suitable husband? According to the books she had read, it was the same with all victims of abuse: they just went out looking for abusive partners. She was determined this was not going to happen to her, however.

"You have to understand," explained Anita, "that he's a bit autistic. I think all men are, actually. They're pretty poor at communicating. For them, communication is a practical thing – a way of getting things done. Look how little time they spend on the phone: no social niceties, just straight to the point. No 'how are you?' just time, date and place, then hang up. Admittedly, Matthew is worse than most, almost Asperger's, I would say, virtually incapable of putting himself in another person's shoes, and really bad with hypothetical situations. That's why it all comes out as so insincere, when he says he loves you. You see, Kate, he has to learn a script. Where the rest of us react instinctively to the wants and needs of others around us, Matthew has to ask himself, how would Anita react to this? He does really love you, but he's pathologically incapable of expressing that love. Okay, he can say the words, but if they are not matched by a kind gesture, or sometimes even the appropriate facial expression, or other body language, his feelings do not come across, so how can you possibly feel loved?"

Matthew figured out some of the reasons why he had always been so judgemental. For one thing, he had consistently avoided the challenges involved in seeking promotion. He had only ever expected to inherit a post once the incumbent was deceased. (As Professor Laurie Taylor used to say in the ***TLS***: 'where there's death, there's hope!') As we know, it was only after he had the authority that went with a promoted post that he started to find himself less inclined to be critical of others. He had managed to learn how to praise his team, and one other big secret relating to control: you only have true control when you feel sufficiently confident to release control. Delegation empowers others without disempowering the delegator.

He learned a valuable piece of advice from a sociologist who was researching the use of personal pronouns. On the face of it, not a riveting topic, but underlying the banality was some powerful information.
"We secretly recorded the telephone conversations of a thousand people, selected to represent socio-economic groupings A to E, and equally representative of males and females. The findings were quite revealing," said Dee.
"Let me guess," pondered Matthew, "Working classes prone to using the third person plural?"
"You're not far wrong, there," said Dee. "Victims' lives are often like that, they see everything that happens in their lives in a passive way. They're fatalistic and rarely see themselves in a position to alter their fate. Consequently, as they are, by definition, not responsible for their own destiny, ***I*** is usually replaced by ***they*** in their sentences, unless they're self-obsessed dependency-culture victims, of course."

"It's remarkable how much you can pick up from all this," said Dee. "There's the subtle inclusiveness of the word, ***we***, for example. Just think how much more difficult it is to go against the implied decision of a meeting, when a speaker uses ***we*** as opposed to ***I.*** You're fighting an army, psychologically speaking, rather than an individual. People that use ***I*** a lot can come across as self-obsessed, self-important – as mavericks, even."
"And what about people that use ***you*** a lot, what's their motivation?" asked Matthew. "That's you, that is," laughed Dee, "That's you all over!"
"I don't follow," said Matthew.
"Well, you wouldn't, would you?" replied Dee, "Thou hypocrite. First remove the beam from thine own eye before thou becomest critical of the moat in thy brother's eye! As you know from your psychology, there's the well-known phenomenon of ***projection***. It's very easy to see failings in another person precisely because you exhibit them yourself, though you're patently unaware of them, of course."

Matthew took some time to reflect on his use of the pronoun, ***you***. Yes, maybe that was a sign of his controlling nature, constantly trying to fix everyone else's life, ***without a thought for himself***, he added, just in some

small way to sweeten the bitter pill that he had just had to swallow. Dee continued,
"Of course, it's a bit of a cliché, I know, but it did transpire that many of the females' chat included the word ***she*** on a recurrent basis, suggesting, no doubt, to all you males that women love to bitch. We're still working on an interpretation of a predilection for ***he*** or even ***it,*** but these were very rare occurrences in our sample, so probably not highly significant."

"Tell you what," said Matthew to Dee, "I'm going to make a concerted effort from now on to default to ***we*** in future – it seems the safest option available."
"You are part of management now, so you had better act accordingly," said Dee, "but don't go talking about yourself in the third person, like senior management have started doing - you know, expressions like: 'I want you to come on board with this new initiative, but do it because you care, not because Joe Bloggs [i.e. ***I***] tell(s) you to do it'. And remember, you have to be ***authentic***: it's no good pretending now, however good an act you could put on."

## Chapter thirty-nine – the actor

When an insane person loses all control over what is right, and allows his imagination to run riot, the immediate casualty – at least from the point of view of the outside world – is the truth. When you are talking to someone in that state of mind, it is very hard to tell whether they are telling the truth or lying: their acting skills are often so convincing.

Matthew started to wonder what happened to people who had been given the wrong diagnosis. He had had several 'Cuckoo's Nest[22]' flashbacks, realising how easily a perfectly sane individual could theoretically become institutionalised. Assuming a good method actor, like himself, wanted to mimic the tell-tale symptoms: The depressive end of the spectrum was quite easy to simulate: all he needed to do was focus on moments of utter despair and his voice would become monosyllabic and his mien lugubrious. The hypomania was harder to achieve. (Perhaps he had always been unipolar, after all?)

At the local herbalist store, he could purchase a packet of St John's Wort. Instead of following the instructions to restrict his intake to a couple per day, he could take the lot in one go – this would generate the desired 'high'. Assuming he had actually carried out this action, he would have experienced a warm glow accompanied by an almost uncontrollable aspiration to rule the world. Money would have been of little interest – indeed, he would happily have stuffed ten-pound notes into the collection-tins of amazed charity volunteers. On the other hand, he would have ranted and raved about the state of the nation and vowed to set his mind to resolving all its social ills. He would have seen great significance in random coincidences; he would have assumed that every celebrity out there would like nothing better than to make his acquaintance because what he had to say was of so earth-shattering consequence.
On seeing such florid displays of megalomania, who would have blamed any self-respecting psychiatrist for diagnosing bipolar? Admittedly, the doctor would have covered all options by appending a question mark after the word 'hypomania'.
---
Alice came over to see Matthew that evening. Alice was not used to this kind of situation, however. ***Little Brother*** had warned her about putting her safety at risk by visiting folk with an unpredictable behaviour pattern. She knew she really should have taken along a colleague, just to be on the safe side. Had she been visiting a female friend with depression, it would not have crossed her mind to arrange for a 'minder', but ***Little Brother*** had counselled her about the potential dangers of mad axe-men. For ever the

[22] One Flew Over The Cuckoo's Nest. Ken Kesey (1962)

risk-taker, Alice decided to go alone to see Matthew, reassuring herself in the knowledge that he would never open up if someone he regarded as a (!!!) accompanied her. Matthew knew instinctively that Alice was (safe).[23]

"How are you?" she asked, unsure how else to open the conversation. After all, that is what you would ask someone who was physically sick - wouldn't you do the same in a case of mental illness?
"Never felt better!" said Matthew, and this was rather disconcerting for Alice. She was taken aback by the unrealistic response, but she felt she had to humour him, just to keep the conversation going.
"But you're ill, aren't you?" confirmed Alice.
"That's for me to know, and for you to wonder about!" responded Matthew, and Alice knew she was going to be drawn into a guessing game, or even to be lured into Matthew's twilight world, where nothing was as it seemed.
"So, are you claiming you're not actually ill?" asked Alice.
"Let's just for one minute dismiss the evidence for me being considered to be ill. Imagine, if you like, that the manic mood was all put on; that the amazingly honest discussion about deviant behaviour was deliberately designed to shock and to prompt action; that the aberrant 'touchy-feely' stuff was just a very good act. Now consider this. How lucid do I seem to you? If you like, I'll engage with you in one of those rational discussions we've always enjoyed, just to let you judge for yourself whether I'm mad, sad, or just plain bad."

Alice was astounded how normal the conversation that followed appeared to be; she just could not say for sure if he was dissembling. Four days later, Matthew's letter arrived, by which time she heard the news from Anita that he had been admitted into a psychiatric unit in England. The letter explained his need to flee south as he did not want to end up in a hospital so far away from everyone he knew. He spent around four weeks inside. That was – at the time - a relatively short stay: most of his fellow- inmates were there for a minimum of six months. Nowadays, shorter stays are more common.
"A bit like the prison population," Alice said to ***Little Brother***, when she next met him with her colleagues over coffee at work. "Not enough accommodation for the number of folk we want to lock up, so we have to let them out on parole much earlier."
"Waste of space," if you ask me, prisons," said ***Little Brother***, "what criminals need is a short, sharp shock."

"You seem to start from the premise that everyone is bad, and in need of correction," said Alice.
"That's right," said ***Little Brother***, "they're all at it, given the chance!"

---

[23] See Appendix (ii)

"I like to come from the opposite position to you," said Alice, "start off, if you like, by seeking out the good in people."
"You'll only end up being disillusioned," said ***Little Brother***.
"But you must admit that everyone responds better to praise than they do to criticism?" said Alice.
"There is absolutely no point in giving praise where it isn't merited," said ***Little Brother***, "no one's allowed to fail a test, nowadays. They even get bonus points to compensate if their hamster died on the date of the examination!"
"I see where you're coming from," said Alice, acknowledging that he did have a valid argument in maintaining that praise should only be given where a student has genuinely risen to the challenge, and achieved their laurels despite tremendous odds against them so doing.

"Do you think we'll be able to trust him with the kids?" asked Bert, Matthew's boss at the college.
"I think it's too much of a risk," said ***Little Brother***, "he might go contaminating them with his funny ideas."
"What about letting him mix with his colleagues?" asked Bert. ***Little Brother*** was concerned,
"I wouldn't like to risk having him alone with a female: you never know, he might be a mad axe-man for all we know, and we have to think about our legal obligations, here. If it can be shown that we haven't taken all reasonable steps to protect his colleagues, the authorities will be down on us like a ton of bricks." Theodora and Matthew had both been going through divorce proceedings prior to his departure, so they had compared notes, particularly on the financial front, and she was puzzled when he did not return to their shared work-space.
"I got far more work down when he was around than I do now with my more talkative female colleagues," she said to Alice.

Hazel reminded the assembled company what a negative impact Matthew's influence had been having on staff morale in recent times.
"He's a real stirrer, that Matthew. Puts dangerous thoughts into people's minds. I think that's what's causing so many folk to take time off with depression. Probably best to put him somewhere where we can keep an eye on him. If only he could learn some ***esprit-de-corps***. He doesn't seem to realise how important it is that management put up a united front."

Hazel was to explore the logic behind this discordant, yet manipulative voice with Matthew later on; but for now it was to be Jean-Paul who helped him examine both the destructive force that negativity can bring with it, as well as the liberating effect it can sometimes generate. The man who 'goes with the flow' often finds himself to have espoused the wrong cause. Expediency can produce short-term gains with horrendous long-term consequences.

## Chapter forty – the dissenter

"You may have been told to avoid the negative," said Jean-Paul, "and to a certain extent, that is true. Negativity is very infectious. Being in the presence of a group of people with a negative, pessimistic, ***feeling-sorry-for-myself*** attitude is hardly an uplifting experience. The person who enters into that atmosphere will always come away feeling intellectually, emotionally and spiritually drained. In a positively-charged atmosphere, on the other hand, you will find people going away invigorated. They will feel noticeably re-energised, mainly due to the fact that everyone present at the encounter had something positive to give: where each person gives, everyone comes away the winner: where most people take, nobody wins, not even the takers, who in the process of draining others of energy, actually drain themselves of it, too."

Matthew could see Jean-Paul's point. He too had often unwittingly drained others of energy and - with hindsight - now understood why they had suddenly started avoiding him like the plague.
"What do you imagine triggered the negativity in you?" asked Jean-Paul.
"Lots of little things, when I look back," said Matthew. "Being a teacher wasn't a good start."
"How do you mean?" asked Jean-Paul.
"However much you know how important it is to praise the little buggers," said Matthew, "if your praise is insincere, they'll pick up on that immediately. To be honest, I never really liked kids, so coming up with a 'Well done!' through clenched teeth was rather unconvincing, to say the least. Added to that, my teaching style was quite heavy on criticism, focussing perhaps unduly on the errors as opposed to the good work. It's not hard to imagine how that work persona carried over into the home environment.

'You don't need to shout!' my son and daughter would say, in unison, when I failed to reduce the level of decibels from the school for a one-to-one encounter in the home.
"I think the closest you'll get to an explanation for your negativity," said Jean-Paul, "is ***projection***. It was yourself whom you were really wanting to criticise for your lack of ambition, and to externalise, if you like, this pent-up emotion, you projected it out onto everyone else. Shall we let your victims elaborate?" Matthew really did want to learn from his mistakes, so he agreed to this somewhat bizarre suggestion.

Anita's voice spoke first:
"Every single talent I had, you would undermine me, usually making me feel that since I couldn't possibly match up to your standard, I should give up."

"I'm truly sorry for that," said Matthew, "It was never intentional, you know."
"I realise that," said Anita, "but I'd have loved to have felt confident enough to continue with my music, just as you have done."
"There's still time, you know," said Matthew, "I used to love hearing you sing the Joni Mitchell songs: I'm getting you a new guitar, right now!"
"Who's next?" asked Jean-Paul.

Kate's voice came through like an apparition hovering between two worlds, "I regret to say that I seem to have inherited your propensity for projection, only I sometimes feel I'm living my life vicariously, as though it really isn't ***my*** life at all. It always feels like regardless of what I achieved, as an athlete or musician, I'll never be a patch on my brother, in your eyes."
"I was always impressed by your achievements, Kate," said Matthew. "You were a fantastic runner and proficient at so many musical instruments; so good, in fact, that the orchestra and sports teams were vying for your contribution. And I just want to tell you now how impressed I was by your absolute lack of fear. Even at primary school, you were doing the so-called ***Irish Crucifix*** on your school residential, deciding that conventional abseiling was far too easy for you and choosing to descend upside-down instead. Can you imagine Mark ever trying something like that?"

"Shall I continue?" asked Jean-Paul.
"No, I think I've got the message, thanks," said Matthew, quickly changing the subject, "you were implying that there may be some forms of negativity that can be productive?" Jean-Paul glanced across at him, in what Matthew took to be a sympathetic manner.
"You'll have heard of the phrase, 'Don't shoot the messenger'? Sometimes, it's important to listen to voices of dissent, so that you do not hurtle head-on into a really bad decision, and when those voices are coming from people who are notorious for their 'it'll never work' mentality, you'll ignore their warnings – because of the person, rather than the message – at your peril."
"Can we do the question-words, again?" asked Matthew, suddenly finding himself propelled back to primary school mode in his infantile request.

"Yes, of course," said Jean-Paul, "***Why not?*** ...You'll have noted that I've started with the one deviation from the norm. Let's see what all the rest have in common, first of all. If you combine any of the remaining question words with a negative, you'll end up with a cautionary suggestion, advocating ***look before you leap***: What not to wear, how not to offend, when not to drink, where not to go after dark, who not to go out with. 'Why not?' on the other hand, reflects a very different proverb, ***nothing ever comes to him who waits***. In fact, it is the awkward question-word, ***why?*** that encourages procrastination, as opposed to risk-taking.

"Then that's helped me decide," said Matthew, "from now on, I'm a ***Y-not***[24] person. No more of that agonising over the pros and cons. No more treading on eggshells to avoid upsetting people because I hadn't considered the consequences. As my colleague, Moira, used to say, 'Don't ask for permission: just do it, and apologise later, if absolutely necessary'. I've finally realised that you can't legislate for everyone else's possible reactions. Everyone I meet nowadays seems to be a control-freak, carefully orchestrating everyone else's entrances, interactions and exits. Why can't we all leave each other alone? If someone takes offence, it's their problem. Folk are just encouraged to blame other people when things go wrong for them, instead of taking responsibility for themselves. I put it down to the compensation culture we have, these days."
"That attitude will really help you achieve your goals," said Jean-Paul. "Now are you absolutely sure that you've shed that negative, controlling characteristic you used to have?" Matthew reflected.
"At least I'll be aware when I feel it coming on," he said.

Jean-Paul decided it was about time for Matthew to be put to the test. For Matthew to finally grow up, he had to stop relying on the crutches that other people – real and imaginary - were providing. So first of all, he had to shed the all-controlling influence of his superego, despite its religious origins.

---

[24] The author acknowledges his indebtedness to the name of Isla's night-club, where he performs with the band.

## Chapter forty-one – the devil

Matthew now had to learn how to grow up. He had spent a whole lifetime being ruled by his ***superego*** which always kept his ***id*** in check. Suddenly liberated from his careful ***what if?*** thinking, Matthew suddenly became aware that there was no longer someone there to police his actions. In Faustian terms, anything that wasn't strictly speaking forbidden, must - by default - be sanctioned. How far would this licence stretch, he wondered?

Some people now state that God is inside every one of us. He's never really been located in one place, anyway. Some used to claim he was omnipresent, though others thought he resided up in the sky somewhere. Some experts in the use of functional magnetic resonance imaging even claim to have identified the so-called 'God-spot' in the brain. Likewise, it might seem logical to assume that the fallen angel, Lucifer, would be located within each individual. After all, we all have our dark side.
"No more Mr Nice Guy!" vowed Matthew, as he resolved to rock the boat more in future.

Although Matthew was enjoying all this mischief, he felt the devil must have a more constructive role to play. Was it not the devil that we have to thank for change? Matthew recalled the old Rolling Stones hit, ***Sympathy for the Devil***, as he strolled through the newly-renamed St Petersburg. You cannot consider ***perestroika*** until after you have blown up a few bridges. Sometimes it is the very act of destruction that creates the possibility of change.

This was not a matter of listening to the fiendish exhortations of some diabolical Mephistopheles. It was an integral part of his own personality that had so long been denied a voice. Okay, sometimes this ***alter ego*** might be ruthless, but he had laudable ends which justified the means.
"You can't make an omelette without cracking a few eggs," he said to himself, but then suddenly felt in need of some reassurance. "Jean-Paul," he called out, "Tell me I'm right, here." There was no response. Just a deathly silence. "That would seem to imply that I'm now on my own," thought Matthew, "Perhaps Jean-Paul is putting me to the test. He wants me to learn how to grow up and take responsibility for my actions, rather than rely on authority figures from the past to censure my every move. I need to cultivate my own moral code. Going against your own moral code is much harder than breaking someone else's rules, like you do if you belong to a strict religion."

"Come on," said Matthew, "Who's going to become the ***advocatus diaboli*** of my alter ego? Jean-Paul is clearly batting for the opposition, it's only right that the other side gets a fair hearing, with an appropriately qualified

advocate." At first his pleas were met with a deafening silence. This situation endured for a matter of months. Then one day in 2001, quite out of the blue, the voluptuous Eve became a significant force in his life.
"Aha!" said Matthew, "So it's true about the devil-woman image: Eve the temptress, and all that."
"Typical misogynous demonization of the female of the species!" interjected the voice of Kate, appearing in his head like a reincarnation of Mary Wollstonecraft.
"Numerologically speaking, the female counts as a ***two***, and that implies duality," said Matthew. Eve tactfully ignored his ***smart-arse*** comments and cut straight to the chase. "If we two are to get along together, we'd better share a bed, sooner rather than later." Matthew was a bit nonplussed by this candour, though he had to admit it was every teenage boy's fantasy to be offered such an invitation from such a delectable ***Mrs Robinson***.
"In your dreams!" mocked the voice of Kate, thinking Matthew must have succumbed to a succubus.
"Is this for real?" he asked Eve, as they climbed into bed.
"Of course it is," replied Eve, "but be discreet: I know your reputation for sharing information, and this would be just too much for some people to take!"

Matthew felt reinvigorated after their encounter; he realised that the future was going to be very bright indeed. He kept the experience very much to himself, but he detected in the close scrutiny of his eyes by some of the ***cognoscenti*** that he was exuding the radiance of a person enjoying a very good sex life.
"You've crossed the line between morality and immorality: do you feel guilty?" asked Eve.
"Not in the slightest," replied Matthew, "I'm a free agent now; we're both adults and nobody's going to get hurt." Eve interpreted this as a good sign, and resolved to pay him visits on future occasions, whenever she felt he was in need of a top-up in his energy levels.

"I thought the succubus was meant to ***drain*** you of energy," commented Kate.
"You're not supposed to know about any of this," said Matthew, "What's the point of me being discreet when you seem to know all about it already?" Kate explained that she had acquired the ability to flit between worlds, ever since that time when she nearly died. Like Matthew, she occasionally straddled two worlds, and sharing her existence in this way meant that she was never quite confined to just one world. Matthew, too, frequently had to drag himself out of what his friends thought was just a form of daydreaming, but, as we know, his dream-world avatar was seriously into doing battle in a parallel universe.

"Let's smoke some dope!" suggested Eve, as they headed out to the beach.

"It's been a long time since I tried Moroccan Gold," said Matthew, "and isn't this stuff much stronger, nowadays?"
"Nothing like the home-grown variety," said Eve, "Totally organic, full-strength, unadulterated (the word was deliberately chosen) shit!" Now, what was it he had learnt about shit? – Oh, yes, that was it, like money, it had to be spread around to do any good. How did that old song from ***Easy Rider*** go? 'Don't bogart that joint, my friend, pass it over to me.' He had to admit that, as a non-smoker, he had missed out on the camaraderie, and could see how, in some perverse way, it contributed to holding together the social fabric of the group. Sharing the weed with Eve, he could swear he was experiencing the taste of apples. He didn't find the ordeal worth the trouble, however, producing, as it did, just one almighty head-ache.

"You prefer it cooked, don't you?" said Eve, "Tell you what, let's bake some hash- cakes to take to the party, and we can sit back and laugh at the effect they have on the guests."
"Seems harmless enough," said Matthew, "perhaps we could take some photos of them as they lose their inhibitions. I might even put my hypnotic skills to use, and get them to do a striptease!"
"Just remember, you have to convince them that it's perfectly normal to get undressed – you need to create the illusion that they are getting ready to take a bath. Then, all you need to do is create in their minds a set of multiple negative hallucinations to disguise the fact that there are lots of people of both sexes in the room, and Bob's your uncle, in next to no time they're cavorting around in the nude!"

"Okay, I'm your catalyst for change," said Eve, "Without me, you'd never get anything done, what with your Health & Safety, your adherence to the rules, your conventional behaviour, and so on. You have to operate at the margins, as Jon used to say. Break some rules. Perfect systems inevitably atrophy. Only dynamic operations are capable of adjusting to constant change. Change is good. Change should be welcomed and embraced wholeheartedly."

What did all this 'catalyst for change' thing mean?

## Chapter forty-two – the lover

When he met Honey in Hull back in 1988, Matthew was finally able to differentiate between love and lust. Only later did he discover how to amalgamate the two successfully. Honey reawakened his sexual desires in a big way, and he was most grateful to her for that experience of renewal. He had resisted the legendary ***seven year itch*** out of loyalty to his equally loyal wife, but the ***fourteen year itch*** came at a time of turmoil in the family, and Honey, he felt, just exploited his vulnerability, though she would presumably have seen things differently. There was potentially a tremendous risk here. Honey's son had been a student in his class. Luckily their carefully arranged encounter coincided with a visit he was making to an individual who was serving an extended period of incarceration, and the two venues were in the same general area.

Honey appealed to him at a purely carnal level; she had clearly planned her seduction technique from the start. On their first meeting, her pink blouse had mysteriously fallen open to reveal a lilac bra – the kind of bra that was not purely of the utilitarian variety. They clawed at each other to remove all clothing as swiftly as possible, going instinctively for sex in the standing position. Matthew's rigidity increased as Honey wrapped her legs around him and their first act was over almost before the prelude had begun. But barely an hour later a return bout was underway, this time ensuring mutual satisfaction. In the background, Matthew heard the radio playing Lionel Ritchie's ***Three Times a Lady***, and rose to the occasion yet again. Oddly enough, the tantric sex he had anticipated never materialised, and sadly, he never heard from or contacted Honey again. It had been a ***one-night-stand*** in many senses of the expression.

Doris, the another one-night-stand, on the other hand, was not so easily forgotten. Having fled to Greece to escape the clutches of the German ***Kripo***[25], Matthew soon discovered she had left him with a memento that took several visits to the special clinic to remove. He was very careful not to engage in sexual relationships during that period for obvious reasons, but his girl-friend at the time seemed to find what she perceived to be his reticence to make love all the more attractive. Not deeming it a wise move to divulge his condition to her, he decided to end the relationship abruptly. After all, that kind of information could spread like wildfire, just like STI's, and would, in the student-world he inhabited, be as good as hanging a bell round his neck and go about screaming out 'Unclean! Unclean!'

"How many partners have you had since your last consultation with me?" enquired the doctor.

---

[25] Criminal Investigation Department

"None at all," replied Matthew, and this was the God's-honest truth.
"Oh, yes," smiled the doctor, "That's what they all say. Just signed up for the monastery, have you?" Seeing another client sitting in the queue, wearing a dog-collar, Matthew felt the ministry was not necessarily such an unusual vocation to cite. "The desperation of celibacy must lead to many priests visiting brothels," he said to the doctor.
"Yes, it's a real shame, because often it really has been just a one-off visit to a prostitute in their case," said the doctor. "Of course, there are some men who sometimes get infected and do not realise it until their partners catch it. One woman told me, when she'd said to her boy-friend, 'thanks for giving me the chlamydia!' that he'd got really annoyed and wanted to know who the cheeky bastard was who had been sending her flowers!"

"Better to come clean," said Matthew, "Maybe I should have told Belinda, and let her decide whether she was prepared to accept someone with an STI. I've always tried to adhere to the motto, ***honesty is the best policy*** – though not for insurance purposes, of course. But what if I've left Doris with an even longer lasting memento?"
"Please explain," replied the doctor.
"One of the human variety: perhaps I've got a son or daughter!" said Matthew.
"I think Doris would have made a greater effort to track you down, if that had been the case," said the doctor, "even if it was only for child maintenance."

There are countless songs that link love and insanity. When you are in love, all rational thought goes out of the window. Comments from colleagues, concerned about his apparent dereliction of duty fell on deaf ears. Love is blind (and deaf, too, so it would seem.) Love encouraged Matthew to be reckless, acting on instinct rather than on common sense. ***Amor vincit omnia***, he thought, suddenly feeling the power that love had to overcome all manner of trials and tribulations. The insanity of love is an entirely different sensation to 'normal' madness. It has one redeeming feature, namely that the quasi-psychosis of a couple in love is generally not only tolerated by society, but actually celebrated and encouraged. Such behaviour, though clearly aberrant, would not lead to them being sectioned, at least not in most civilised countries.

"I know Saint Paul comes across as a bit of a misogynist," said Matthew, "Though his thoughts on the overwhelming power of charity are clear. Faith and hope may be important, but not as important as ***love*** which has a more enduring characteristic. Of course, it has only been during the last century that the decision was taken to substitute the word ***charity*** for ***love***."
"Maybe Paul should have written a letter to the ***Philadelphians***, in addition to the ones to the Corinthians," said Anita.

"You're one ahead of me there," said Matthew, inwardly kicking himself for failing to get the allusion.
"Brotherly love," explained Anita, "perhaps he wasn't into heterosexual love at all."
"That's where the theologians have a problem: words never translate perfectly. For example, ***erotic*** comes from Eros, the Greek god of love, but ***amorous*** comes from Amor, or Cupid. The derived meanings are never interchangeable," said Matthew.
"Next thing I know, you'll be challenging one of the basic tenets of my Catholic faith," said Anita.

"I suppose I ***should*** target Peter, since you've had a go at Paul," said Matthew, "but I think I'll choose Mary, just for the sake of sexual equality, of which I know you're an advocate. Take that 'virgin birth' confabulation. It was probably based on a mixture of borrowed ideas from other faiths and notions that got lost in translation. The Latin word, ***virgo***, literally translates as maiden – it doesn't necessarily imply ***virgo intacta***."
"You lapsed Protestants," retorted Anita, "Always so keen to point out that we worship graven images. At least, we don't have a ***pick-and-mix*** religion like yours!"

The role of the lover had been a truly liberating experience; but for the present, in the confines of the psychiatric hospital, all he could do was dream.

**Chapter forty-three – the dreamer**

It is a paradox that we can be at once dismissive of dreamers as poor deluded souls living a ***Walter Mitty*** like existence, and yet at the other extreme look up to them as visionaries such as Martin Luther King. Like the fine line between genius and madness, the distinction between a shrewd business idea and a delusory notion can, like beauty, be purely in the eye of the beholder. Many talented ***messengers*** have been shot down in this way: there was nothing wrong with their dream. Either they went about selling their dream in the wrong way and alienated crucial potential benefactors, or they were not prepared to persevere after some initial setbacks and rejections.

Matthew had a lot of time to think in the hospital. It was at times like that, when the world had taken away from him every scrap of power and influence he had ever had, that, strangely enough, he imagined he was omnipotent. His ability to rule the world seemed self-evident; his degree of influence over world leaders and major celebrities indisputable. He totally rejected any notion that he might be suffering from delusions of grandeur: he had always known he was Jesus Christ; it was just that now he was going to perform a few miracles in order to prove the fact.

Perhaps his childhood exposure to religion had first generated that angelic behaviour that his music teacher held up as a model to his fellow pupils. Obviously, this led to him being universally vilified by the class, rather than, as the music teacher had naively imagined, emulated for his good behaviour. As a student, he actually looked like many of the biblical images of Christ, with his full beard, long hair and sandals, and student friends would jokingly ask him to perform miracles, like turning the water into wine.
"Go on, Jesus," taunted one devilish student, "show us how you walk on water!" Matthew paused at the edge of the water, then started making his way further out to sea, whereupon he promptly sank.
"It's not quite so easy when you have holes in your feet!" he explained.

Always on the look-out for coincidences, as we know, Matthew had, in 1967, attended a concert by the Strawberry Hill Boys, who were later to become more famous as the Strawbs. They sang a song entitled, 'He was the Man who called himself Jesus', and somehow Matthew knew that one day, he too would experience such an alleged indicator of insanity.

Had he kept to ***one*** celebrity persona, people might just have been able to suspend disbelief for an instant, and enter into his world. It was clearly a world where good forces predominated. Yet the very next instant, he was Superman, Nostradamus or some other kind of latter-day superhero, and hence very difficult to follow or indulge. Does a visionary would-be entrepreneur differ so greatly from a crazy delusionary? It would appear to be purely a matter of degree.

In order to achieve his or her ambitions, the wheeler-dealer has to operate at the margins, often outside of the law, certainly in the early stages of his or her career. If he is lucky, the State will turn a blind eye to his juvenile peccadilloes and give him a knighthood. You never thrive, if you are obsessed with Health and Safety issues.. When he was on a visit to Russia, Matthew observed how quickly the young movers and shakers became millionaires. Not being obsessed by safety, they are not hamstrung by our risk-averse culture, and indeed have taken what might be seen as an unfair advantage in being able to cut corners, exploiting their compatriots, as well as, increasingly, immigrant labour to obtain great financial rewards. Sometimes mad, hare-brained schemes do work.

"Madness is the closest thing to genius," said Matthew to Dave, his room-mate in the psychiatric hospital, and thought for a while how unfair it was that society never takes any chances with 'mad' people. "Maybe, if they let us, we could actually solve some global problems, because we have a different way of looking at the world. When I am manic, I feel like Saul, in the sense that I have had a Damascene revelation, as if the scales have been peeled away from my eyes. I can see, not just the veneer of a situation, but almost like Röntgen with his X-rays, I can penetrate into other people's deepest thoughts. It's like telepathy, in a way – though I can get ***that*** occurring on a normal day, especially with close friends or family."

Dave agreed,
"Take Jesus," he began, "arriving here on Earth for his second coming, they'd have him locked up almost before he uttered a word. He'd have to dissemble, at least for about forty years, in order to hoodwink the people into believing in him. Now that Barack Obama fellow, he could be Jesus, you'd never know, would you? Not at all the stereotypical Messianic figure with delusions of grandeur, is he? Seems quite self-effacing, for a potential presidential candidate. No doubt about his charisma, though. Radiates out, even from TV and newspaper photographs. Must be genuinely awesome to meet him in person. Best part about it is, if he actually were Jesus, he could eventually be in a position to save the world: no one's going to challenge the President. He'll just have to keep quiet on the religious front. None of that evangelising. He's deliberately left that ambiguous, though: he might even be a Muslim, for all I know."
"He's got all the I's," said Matthew, "Intelligence, Imagination, Integrity, Idealism: he's immaculate, imperturbable, impressive, inclusive, indefatigable, independent-minded, instinctive and intuitive; probably one of the Illuminati, too, I wouldn't wonder."

Matthew found Barack Obama to be quite unusual for a presidential hopeful. Like Matthew, he had had to learn how to function as an interloper, but unlike Matthew, he had the additional issue of race to contend with. So far as Matthew was aware, Obama was an incredibly well-balanced individual, given his history. On the other hand, as a classic case of bipolar disorder, Matthew swung dramatically from depression to elation and then back down again. First of all, we see a glimpse of the nadir before we look at the zenith.

## Chapter forty-four – the depressive

The term ***depression*** has its origins in the circulatory system. Apparently, it was initially used to describe low blood pressure, or hypotension. Matthew occasionally, very occasionally, plumbed the depths of despair, but combining his birth sign (Virgo) with his Chinese sign (the rat), it was perhaps not surprising that he had a penchant for subterranean passages in the labyrinth of the subconscious mind. It is to gain an insight into the ***depressive*** end of the bipolar condition that we get to observe the nadir of his experiences, very rarely seen in public. Thereafter, we shall get the opportunity to see the zenith which bipolars are happier to display to the world.

It was a dark, dismal day in December, (alliteration to compensate for the lack of vitamin D), and Seasonal Affected Disorder was common at this latitude. Matthew kept his own chart on the calendar to map expected highs and lows on his bipolar cycle, so he anticipated that this particular depression would start to lift in a couple of days. Solitude is probably the worst companion to depression. It was Christmas Day 2001 out there in the real world and Matthew was well aware how such artificially created high-points of the year can trigger suicidal thoughts in those particularly susceptible. Because he knew that he would be spending Christmas alone, he had deliberately ignored the build-up to the big day. In fact, come to mention it, in retrospect he had always tried to chicken out - or should we say ***turkey*** out - of Christmas and other holidays, preferring instead to take on part-time work such as driving taxis. Clearly, this had been a coping strategy: if he avoided potential highs, the lows would not seem too bad in contrast. In fact, he liked to think that he maintained what he called a ***flat*** existence which quite effectively ironed out all the peaks and troughs.

"Need a little cheering up?" asked Jean-Paul. "You seem somewhat distraught." At times like these, Matthew sought the solace of Latin.
"Dum spiro, spero[26]," he said. Jean-Paul was gratified by this response,
"I'm glad to hear you've fought off those suicidal thoughts," he said. "Now remembering what Paul says, ***love*** will be your salvation, ultimately, but in the meantime, hope and faith will see you through. And now, before I give you the details, I want you to promise me never to share with anyone what I am about to tell you. Will you make me that promise?"
"Yes, of course," agreed Matthew, "You have been my constant guide throughout my darkest times, how could I refuse to keep such a promise?"

There followed an elaborate series of revelations, culminating in one amazing secret, and to this day, Matthew has stuck to his guns and never

---

[26] If you're still breathing, then there's hope.

shared its details; nor is he about to now. Suffice it to say that the way he took in the information was like a spy just handed his instructions on a sheet of edible rice-paper who promptly consumes his ***vade-mecum*** to destroy the evidence. In his head, he carefully folded up the set of instructions, over and over again, until the resulting origami puzzle became sufficiently small as to fit into one of the deep recesses of his subconscious mind. The instant he took that step, he knew he was back on the road to recovery. It felt like the worries of the world had been lifted from his shoulders and he handed them back to Atlas where they belonged.

"You're very quiet today, Matthew," said Anita, "Should I be worried? This usually indicates an imminent depressive phase." Matthew forced himself to communicate, "Just pensive, that's all." That was about the sum total of his utterances for the day. Although he had only been up for two hours, he went straight back to bed and stayed there till tea-time, only surfacing a couple of times to go to the toilet. Anita ended up posing rhetorical questions since no responses were forthcoming,
"Is it the depression that makes you want to sleep, or is the excessive amount of sleep that makes you depressed?" she wondered. Even after tea, when they sat down to watch what Matthew would under normal circumstances have deemed to be an interesting film, he dosed off again half way through it.
"Who's that character?" he asked on awakening, having literally lost the plot.
"We're onto a different film, now," said Anita, "the one you were watching finished half an hour ago!"

Despite being rather distant for much of the time, Matthew clearly benefited from social interaction during such phases. If he had still been living alone, his condition would have got much worse.
"What can I do to get you to snap out of it?" asked Anita, feeling that there must be something that could break the spell.
"Just let it take its course," said Matthew, "Anyway, I think human beings ought to hibernate at this time of year."

Matthew and Anita watched a documentary on TV about a girl with two heads who was to undergo an operation to remove (i.e. kill) her twin.
"She might survive to have a near-normal and fulfilling life without her twin attached to her head, but I keep asking myself who the operation is for: is it for the girl, or the society that does not find two-headed freaks in any way aesthetically pleasing. The two faces are like the two masks that have come to symbolise comedy and tragedy, and guess which one the doctors decided to sacrifice?"
"I don't think I can bear to see that face any longer," said Anita, knowing that the poor creature would be terminated once the doctors blocked her access to the oxygenated blood that she and her twin-sister shared.

"Look at that tormented facial expression," said Matthew. "She doesn't appear to be able to make any other expression than a frown." Just then the two heads turned, and they caught sight of the other twin, smiling at the camera. "I think God is trying to tell us something," said Matthew.
"Oh, really, said Anita. "And why would he want to create such an aberration?" Matthew explained his thinking,
"We need misery in order to appreciate joy," he said. "Imagine the sense of loss this smiling young girl's going to feel as she grows up. She'll probably feel guilty, too; guilty that her sister had to be killed so that she could enjoy the indulgence of life."

"Wouldn't it be great if we could be happy all the time?" asked Anita.
"No," replied Matthew, without hesitation. "That would be Huxley's ***Brave New World*** where they abolished the slings and arrows of outrageous fortune. All I would say is, 'if you're happy and you know it, see a shrink.' If you ***were*** happy all the time, you'd be living in a fantasy world. The real world requires a much more balanced reaction: sometimes joy; sometimes sadness. All part of life's rich tapestry, as they say." Anita was disappointed with his response. She had hoped he would share her dream.
"So how do you live with the lows?" she asked.
"I know it's a hackneyed old saying, but life is like a roller-coaster, so you know that however bad things are at the moment, they can always get better."
"Wasn't that New Labour's slogan?" asked Anita, with a wry smile.
"Even politicians eventually have to admit you can't avert the inevitable ***depression!***" said Matthew.

"Another trick," said Matthew, "is to exploit depression in a creative way. Playing the bass guitar, I am regularly exposed to low frequency sounds. Perhaps that explains why most bass players look sad. But then, I find ***the blues*** tends to generate some good musical compositions, and wallowing in the misery paradoxically induces a mild euphoria." Anita nodded in agreement,
"Wasn't it the Epicureans who wallowed in their emotions?" Matthew certainly preferred their philosophy to the old stiff-upper-lip attitude of the Stoics, but by his interpretation of their philosophy, the Epicureans were always in pursuit of happiness, and he tended to prefer the hedonistic search for pleasure:

> ***Happiness is hard to get, pleasure – that's easy;***
> ***But don't come to me, if you don't see my hedonistic philosophy, baby!***

***JS/1968***

"When you're really down, what's it like?" asked Anita.

"It's difficult to be objective, of course, because the whole experience is so self-indulgent, you fail to get any sort of perspective on it, but it's like your other self is the child again, being unjustly punished, and you get to empathise with that child so closely, you burst into tears. It's not yourself you're crying for: it's that poor kid – maybe he or she was you in another life."

"The psychiatrists tell you to rewrite the script," said Anita.
"What?" said Matthew, "and pretend your past never happened, I suppose? It's a good idea to leave the past behind, locked away, if you like, but still there to be accessed at some future date, if necessary. Remember, we are the sum-total of our memories. Don't let the psychiatrists erase them, like they did with that woman in St Thomas's hospital. All that sleep-therapy took away so much of her memory; she can't even recall having given birth to her children."

"But you haven't really told me what it's like when you're down," said Anita. Matthew remembered an analogy from his old friend, Graham:
"it's like trying to walk through treacle".
"A kind of inertia?" asked Anita.
"Yes," said Matthew.
"And what's it like when you're really high?" asked Anita.
"Fantastic!" said Matthew, without hesitation. "Perhaps I just need to raise my blood pressure, or play a high frequency musical instrument in order to induce euphoria."

## Chapter forty-five– the maniac

***Hypomania***, on the other hand, is a mixed blessing. Matthew relished that sense of 'arousal' it gave him, but the very fact that it made him ***out of control*** made him dangerous at that vulnerable time.

"Could be cyclothymia," said Suggs, the psychiatrist. Incidentally, Suggs was quite an accomplished jazz flautist, so potentially Matthew was to have some common ground with him, playing as he later did in a traditional jazz band.
"Look," said Matthew, "I've ***not*** been sectioned, I came voluntarily - however reluctantly - but I'm here, all the same. Personally, I can't see what all the fuss is about. I've never felt better."
"But you're not yourself," said Anita.
"Maybe that's not the self I want to be any more," said Matthew.
"You threw a beer-mat at me," said Anita, "and I can't cope with all that frenetic activity, as you pace the floor and rearrange the furniture every night."
"So my euphoria is illusory, is it?" Matthew asked the psychiatrist.
"You may perceive your hypomania as a good mental state to reside in. We don't," said the psychiatrist, and promptly prescribed suitable sedatives.
"So the treatment's about making life easier for everyone else, not taking my views into consideration at all?" said Matthew.
"Your behaviour verges on the bizarre," said the psychiatrist. "You're in no fit state to be able to make any rational assessment of your thinking at present."

For a brief spell, Matthew had felt really alive for once in his life. So what if he did start spending money, for a change. He had always been a notorious skinflint, according to his drinking-partners, but now he was buying rounds of drinks, quite liberally.
"Slow down, Matthew," his pal, Kenny had said, "you're too fast for me. Tell me the joke again." But now the 'racing thoughts' were taking over. You could always tell by the state of Matthew's handwriting – which was pretty well illegible at the best of times - if he was going through a hypomanic interlude. His hand just could not keep up with his brain and the poor addressee witnessed a mysterious shorthand that even Matthew occasionally could not decipher.

"I've never seen him manic, or even hypomanic, before," said Anita.
"The medication will help him learn how to control the highs and lows," said Carys, the Mental Health Officer, who coincidentally happened to be an acquaintance of Anita's. Matthew remembered Carys from before. She had bright orange hair, hippy clothes and a hypnotic voice. When he met

her ***on the outside*** along with Anita at a dinner-party, she was dabbling in the occult, and reading tarot cards.
"Nothing should upset him any more, so he won't get depressed; but, equally, it won't allow him to get too elated, either."
"I've seen him quite high at parties and other celebrations," said Anita.
"Alcohol is strictly off-limits," replied Carys. "And I wouldn't let him go anywhere near recreational drugs. He just doesn't need any form of artificial stimulation to achieve even mild euphoria."
"Are you sure he is ill?" asked Anita.
"I think if you'd seen the way he behaved in hospital, ranting and raving, you'd have been left in no doubt," replied Carys. "Personally, I think he's way off the scale on the paranoid-schizoid continuum."

"We will have to keep those delusions of grandeur in check," said Dr Sugar.
"They're not delusions," responded Matthew, "I am really charismatic now; haven't you noticed my halo?" Matthew did have a strange glow about him, rather like a novice runner who has just finished his first marathon, or a someone who spent too long under a sun-lamp, though the overall effect was more repulsive rather than attractive to the outside world, and his attempts to communicate with strangers were met with embarrassment rather than engagement on their part.

"Do you think he should be driving a car?" asked Anita.
"Better inform DVLA," said Doctor Suggs. "He'll get it back when he's no longer perceived to be a risk." What he did not mention was the difficulties Matthew would experience subsequently. 'Have you ever suffered from mental illness?' was one of the questions on the form you had to complete if you wanted to hire a car or van. Then there was the small matter of insurance: what happened to the no claims bonus if there was an extended period where the policy holder did not drive a car? Equally challenging was getting your licence back after such episodes.

Matthew had to learn how to be an effective liar, just to survive in this changed environment, where he was no longer in control. That was, in effect, how he learned to dissemble and dissimulate sufficiently well as to avoid having to take his medication.

## Chapter forty-six– the liar

***"Lies, damned lies and statistics"***

***Disraeli***

Leading up to his 'voluntary' spell in the psychiatric hospital in the year 2000, Matthew felt an uncontrollable desire to communicate in writing, ideally with people who had clout. Of course, his manic state of mind ensured that most of his communications ended up relegated to the waste paper bin, since they totally dispensed with all the necessary formalities. Not only did they ignore the conventions applied when writing to people of status, they added insult to injury by the fact that they were written in red ink (actually orange because that was now the colour of choice for Matthew) and reinforced with copious quantities of punctuation, notably exclamation marks. (E-mailers call it shouting).

"Do you promise to tell the truth, the whole truth and nothing but the truth?" asked the judge.
"I do," said Matthew, knowing that all along, his answers would prove to be ***economical with the truth***, in parliamentary language. Like politicians, he had learned how to spin information, hardly ever attempting to answer the question posed, but coming with his own agenda of items that he wanted to make sure he got across. Jean-Paul joined the debate,
"What ***is*** a lie, Matthew?" Matthew knew at once that there was not going to be a simple answer to this question, but he felt he had a reasonable starting-point.
"It depends who you're lying to. If it's to yourself you are lying, that's one thing; if it's to other people, it may be deliberate or it may be unintentional."

Jean-Paul offered a way forwards,
"Do you regret telling family secrets to Kate and Mark? You realise how much it upset them at the time. What need was there for revealing that information?"
"No need whatsoever," replied Matthew. "I just felt an uncontrollable urge to tell the truth, regardless of the consequences. I suppose I had discovered the power of the truth in beating my alleged superiors who had only been able to come up with a web of lies in response. Even though they had carefully rehearsed the script from their hymn sheets, it was gratifying to find that the truth always prevailed, effectively demolishing their arguments." Jean-Paul warned him to go easy with this newly-discovered weapon:
"Discretion, Matthew, discretion. There are times when it's right to speak up, but other times where it's in the best interests of all concerned to remain silent."

"Money is the root of all evil," said Jean-Paul. "You can't serve God and Mammon, so it says in the Bible." Matthew agreed,
"I think the devil must have been an economist."
"Please clarify," said Jean-Paul.
"Well, he must have been the first ***soul trader***; probably the only one, come to think of it," said Matthew.
"And do you feel you sold your soul to the devil, Matthew?" asked Jean-Paul.

"Only small fragments of it," said Matthew, drawing an analogy with the defragmentation process. "I had to free up some space in my head, so I thought I'd let him have the crap – you know, the equivalent of clutter in your home: redundant ideas saved up for a rainy day that is realistically never going to arrive; resentment at being passed over for promotion; hurt from having been treated shabbily; envy at others' perceived successful careers (usually measured in financial terms); frustration at missed opportunities, etc, etc. But I realise I may end up in limbo, as a result of all this purging. Partial defragmentation is like being in a cleft stick: no way forwards and no way back."

"So what you're saying is you've signed over all the negative stuff?" asked Jean-Paul. "Of course," said Matthew, "Give the devil his due, that's what I say. Those parts of my soul I could cheerfully do without - they were weighing me down. Now I feel liberated. I can start anew without being obstructed by demons from the past. I should have dealt with them at the time – I realise that now. It was part of my character to procrastinate, even if it was just a simple thing like replying to letters."

"And you were able to do a deal with him in which you jettisoned all that baggage," said Jean-Paul. "The devil's there, inside your head, and he attaches himself to all your self-doubt, cynicism, scepticism, sloth, boredom, hatred, envy, etc. With the body, it's relatively simple to get rid of garbage, because we take in nutriment, and excrete what we don't need, but with the brain, the process seems to be contaminated by the fact that too much goes in and not enough comes back out again. Mentally ill patients should learn to flush the faeces from their brains."

"That's the nice thing about computers," said Matthew. "Garbage in – garbage out. At least it does come out again. The best therapy is to express all your personal garbage in words. Probably, it's preferable to write it down, in a diary, a poem or a book – that way, you're not bending every poor soul's ear with your worn-out gramophone record, and possibly contaminating them into the bargain. I know some counsellors come away from their psychotherapy sessions feeling positively – or more accurately negatively - drained."

"Now," said Jean-Paul, "back to the defragmentation process. From all these tiny fragments, I want you to identify which characteristics go together to form the essential ***you***." Matthew was at a bit of a loss, faced with the mountain of splinters, and asked Jean-Paul for assistance. "Try concentrating on the elements you don't like about your personality," he said. Matthew began to sift through the fragments of glass; but they cut his fingers to shreds every time he had to discard any single one of them. "You're still having problems with your filing system, aren't you?" said Jean-Paul, "You're going to have to be much more ruthless. No more access to the 'pending' tray for you. Put them all for recycling, if you like – you'd be surprised how helpful other people might find the characteristics that you yourself despise."

## Chapter forty-seven – the assassin[27]

"The judge didn't say I was being tried for a crime I had committed," said Matthew. "He said 'a crime I was ***going to*** commit' and linked it to my anger." Jean-Paul waxed philosophical again,
"Have you ever asked yourself, if it came to the ultimate choice, how you would commit suicide?" asked Jean-Paul.
"I thought even the thought of such a deed was taboo amongst religious types such as you?" replied Matthew.
"It's just a philosophical point. It could give you an insight into your motivational thoughts," said Jean-Paul.

"Well," said Matthew, "I don't like the idea of distressing my relatives and friends unduly, and I wouldn't want to give the authorities unnecessary hassle, like having to look for my body, pick up the pieces, or retrieve it from some godforsaken ravine. So that would rule out my preferred exit routes: driving off a cliff at high speed or jumping from a plane at high altitude.
"Would your death have to be such a macho one?" enquired Jean-Paul.
"Interesting thought, that one," said Matthew, "I suppose by the time you decide to end it all, you shouldn't really be worrying about whether your chosen manner of suicide is 'cool' or not. Nevertheless, an overdose does strike me as more of a female exit strategy."

Matthew continued, "Perhaps the ideal self-sacrificing way to go would be to volunteer for bomb-disposal work, but there's always the chance that I'd survive against all the odds and that would kind of defeat the whole purpose, at least from my personal point of view." Jean-Paul offered a solution,
"you could, of course, exit this life the way we put down animals, using muscle relaxants?"
"When I watched an animal die in that way, it seemed to be putting up quite a fight to survive. Anyway, this is a pointless discussion, because I just wouldn't do it. I'd rather kill someone else," said Matthew.
"Precisely," said Jean-Paul. "I was hoping you would say that. Now, who is it that you hate enough to want to kill him or her?"

Matthew could not answer this question,

---

[27] Hashshashin were eaters of hashish. During the Crusades, assassins intoxicated themselves on the drug prior to committing their deadly deed.

"I feel my anger is directed against so much in the world that it's become too diluted. I cannot focus on any one individual. Murder is often fuelled by alcohol and sober people like me do not generally commit murder."
"But if I were to suggest to you, as a would-be assassin, that smoking a joint would give you sufficient ***Dutch Courage*** to kill someone, would you believe me?" asked Jean-Paul. Matthew used to dismiss the link between taking cannabis and mental illness, but latterly he began to see that the purer home-grown version, ***skunk***, often induced violent impulses in some of his acquaintances.
"You only have to look into their eyes, when they've taken this new stuff, and you can see where their thoughts are leading them," he said.

Then Jean-Paul tried to get Matthew to make a contrast,
"Anger's not like love, you know. The more people you share ***love*** with, the better it is for all concerned." Matthew questioned the veracity of this premise,
"I believe that you can only admit to loving a limited number of people. Otherwise the love seems diluted to a trickle of worthless sentimental effusiveness."

Jean-Paul acknowledged that, occasionally, some people got the wrong idea of what love really is. "There are those who are under the misguided impression that their love can be extended to whole countries of people, and some even think they can empathise with the suffering of bygone civilisations." Matthew agreed. "I love my family, but I wouldn't say I love my friends, except the really close friends, and I couldn't possibly go beyond my parents and grandparents to embrace notions of some kind of atavistic love."

"Let's examine those impulses you've been getting recently," said Jean-Paul.
"It used to be spikes," said Matthew. "Spikes advancing towards my eyes. I had to cover my eyes to protect them whenever I got an image of the spikes."
"Come on, Matthew, concentrate," said Jean-Paul, "I'm asking you about the ***present***, not the past." Matthew shrugged his shoulders,
"I don't really see there's any difference. Time's an artificial concept." Jean-Paul persisted:
"The thoughts, Matthew, the thoughts you've been having."
"Oh, yes," said Matthew, starting to focus on the disturbing ideas that kept coming into his head.

"It's all about ***splitting***. The axe needs to fall exactly in the middle of the forehead. Incidentally, do psychiatrists still cut through the ***corpus callosum*** to improve patients' behaviour? Perhaps that's what lies at the heart of the problem: redundant associations between the left and right

hemispheres." Jean-Paul ignored Matthew's diversionary tactics, and pursued the mention of the skull-splitter.
"Why the axe, Matthew?" Matthew smiled,
"***Little Brother*** must have tipped you off. Gives you a splitting headache, incidentally, the cleaver. Funny, how management like to wield it to get rid of what they call the ***dead wood***."

Jean Paul, as we know, wanted to help Matthew to defragment his soul, and therefore set Matthew off in a direction diametrically opposed to splitting.
"So what's the opposite of split?" Matthew consulted the linguist within him. "Marriage," came the reply.
"I'm looking for something a little broader than that," said Matthew.
"How about 'unity' or 'union'?" suggested the linguist.
"No, that's not working, either," said Matthew. "I believe I may have to cross the divide, and – horror of horrors - ask a scientist."
"How about Fusion?" asked the voice of the nuclear physicist.
"Exactly," responded Matthew, the scientist manqué, who had now arrived at his solution.

The geneticist's voice chimed in with the physicist's earlier comment, drawing Matthew's attention to the way life begins when one cell splits into two,
"But, of course, we haven't yet learned how to reverse that process, so I can't give you a suitable analogy for the process you are attempting to achieve." The economist stepped in, talking about mergers, synergies and vertical integration,
"Big is beautiful. Globalisation is the only way forward. It cuts out the inconvenience of having to comply with petty national legislation."
"Any excuse to cook the books!" said the cook, but then he offered Matthew a metaphorical fruitcake, an ***Apfelstrudel*** in turmoil.

"All these tiny fragments of your personality, Matthew," said the cook, "they're like the ingredients of your personality. Leave any single one of them out, vary the proportions and the result's a disaster. The mix has to be perfect: neither too dry, nor too moist." Matthew was delighted,
"I can really relate to that," he said. "But how does the oven fit in?" The cook explained.
"The oven represents your brain. Whether you put your God-given talents to good use or hide them under a bushel is up to you."
"How am I doing so far?" asked Matthew.
"Not bad," said the cook, "Trouble is, you're so impetuous. You ***are*** an ideas-man, but to put it bluntly, the ideas have a tendency to come out half-baked. Let them stew a little longer before you submit them to public scrutiny."

Matthew approached the ghost writer.

"Do you think some of these characters need to be eradicated? Is it a bit heavy on anonymous stereotypes?" Professor Lucy Stevenson suggested he consult with the newspaperman,
"Journalists have always been rather good at ***character*** assassinations." Matthew had not thought about destroying reputations before, but he had seen the results,
"That's what you folk from the media do," said Matthew to Andrea. "You build up these nobodies with the promise of fame and fortune, only to relish their practically inevitable downfall."
"Personally, I think we're ***very*** responsible in the way we treat members of the public," said Andrea.
"***Some*** of you are, when we remind you that mental illness has to be handled sensitively," said Matthew.
"So what do ***you*** think causes these fame-hungry individuals to crack up?" she asked.

Matthew launched forth.
"Talent shows encourage folk to lose their identity, to reject the very characteristics that made them what they are, and replace these with pseudo-personalities the sponsors have invented for them to inhabit. It's hardly surprising that they start to fail to be able to distinguish between reality and fantasy. This whole celebrity thing is just one big con," said Matthew.
"And does that include politicians?" asked the journalist.
"Well," said Matthew, "just observe the manic look in their eyes. Their megalomania is fed by euphoria which in turn stems from the aphrodisiac nature of the power they have assumed."

"And what about the wealthy?" asked the economist. Matthew had observed a gradual but steady decline generated by redundancies in the financial services. "Marriages are breaking up in the City, because wives cannot accept the loss of status engendered by their husbands' demotion or change of occupation. Many cannot adjust to an income that would represent an absolute fortune to the average ***woman-in-the street***."
"But we must get them spending again to keep the retail trade afloat," said the economist, "We can't afford for them to stop buying clothes with their credit cards." Matthew sighed,
"Maybe that's why the world's in such a sorry state: too much credit."

"I think you're demonising half the population," said Frank, the priest, "why are you so critical of the world?"
"Because so many aspects of the way we live are based, if you'll excuse the expression, on crap ideas," said Matthew. "Now, I understand that life has to be a struggle. Competition and cooperation do not necessarily have to be mutually exclusive ideals. What I find repulsive is the way folk are persuaded to part with their hard-earned cash in exchange for crap. The

latter is usually a so-called 'product' that preys on their fears: insurance, health, peer pressure, finance or legal services. Otherwise, it might be an advertisement encouraging them to believe that by changing their appearance they can change their identity and gain the respect of their peers."

"You are starting to disintegrate," said the priest. "You must remember to preserve your integrity at all costs." Matthew expressed his gratitude to the priest for offering him a survival strategy.
"Throughout my ordeal I have been able to say that I always sought out the truth." The priest agreed,
"If we disregard occasional bouts of fragility, which were predictable in the circumstances, I think we can safely say that you have acted throughout with integrity, honesty and probity. Now that you have effectively exorcised all the demons who have been running your life, you'll be able to start afresh. But we don't want them to go infecting other poor souls: I suggest you get the archivist to help you put them into some semblance of order. You'd better have them all framed to be on the safe side - just to stop them framing you for their assassination, you understand".

# *Episode III*

## Chapter forty-eight – the cyclist

**Mens sana in corpore sano**
**Juvenal 10, 356**

Matthew had, up until the time of his breakdown, always had a tendency to be ***reactive***. From now on, he decided, he was going to be more ***proactive***. It was now summer 2000: six months on from his breakdown. There were things he needed to change about the way he had been living his life, both for the wider good of mankind, and, coincidentally, just out of enlightened self-interest. But first of all, he had to find a way of challenging the 'label' that the medical profession had given him.

Having a record of psychiatric illness, the attitude with which you are confronted by your G.P. is usually one that dismisses any physical symptoms that you may allege you are suffering from.
"Feeling a little depressed, are we?" suggested Dr Martin.
"***You*** may be, but I'm reasonably chipper," replied Matthew, "but if you don't mind, would you have a look at this rash, please?"

"He's walking in a very odd way," commented ***Little Brother***, when Matthew returned to his work. "Do you think he's heading for another episode, Alice?"
"If he has any more episodes, he'll be on his way to making a serial!" joked Alice, realising that Matthew would by now have worked out a pun on the homonym, thanks to the invention of Doctor Kellogg. When Alice, resuming her role as Matthew's confidante, asked Matthew if everything was okay, he divulged the fact that he was actually suffering from shingles and found it quite uncomfortable when walking. "Better get the G.P. to confirm that, just to allay suspicions," advised Alice.
"Already have," beamed Matthew, "you can have a look at the rash if you don't believe me!" Alice tactfully declined this invitation, taking him at his word. "I've still got the propensity to gravitate to the right hand side of corridors, of course, because the stroke put me a bit off-balance. My facial muscles seem to be back to normal now, though. Sometimes I get a little aphasia from time to time, but only if I have to say ***haloperidol*** !"
"Our mutual friend, Jimmy, always recommended cycling: it might help with your balance," said Alice.
"Yes, and it was Jimmy that started me back on cycling, thirty years after I thought I'd given it up for good. I'll certainly give it a try," replied Matthew.

His first attempts were comical, like someone trying to ride home after becoming inebriated, or like a scene from a silent movie, but gradually he managed to steer in a straight line and took up the 'loops', as Jimmy called them, that took no longer than one hour to complete. Folk with psychiatric conditions can generally benefit from walking, but the very thought of encountering a stranger who might make an attempt to engage you in conversation will often deter them from going out. You'll find them booking a taxi to take them a hundred yards to avoid having to pass by people on the street and have to make eye-contact.

Cycling is different. Yes, you will still encounter people on your travels, but the encounters are necessarily brief, perhaps accompanied by a nod of the head, smile or the occasional 'hi!' Then you are off on the road again, hoping you do not get a puncture, if you happen to be on the pessimistic end of the spectrum of bipolar at the time. The exercise is gentle, but can be cranked up a little to strengthen the heart muscles. For reasons of safety, you cannot do as much thinking as you can with walking, but if you choose a quiet road, there is still plenty of room for day-dreaming.

Matthew had always wondered why psychiatric patients were often described as unbalanced or unstable. It was only when he tried out the equipment in the gymnasium that he found himself unable to balance on the piece of apparatus designed with precisely that skill in mind. It basically consisted of a ball attached to a board. He remembered once trying out a trick-bike where the front wheel turned to the left whenever you steered it to the right, and vice-versa. You probably needed to be a psychiatrist (trick-cyclist) to ride it!

The imbalance had returned after the stroke, and he found himself unusually attracted to right wing candidates when it came to the General Election. Previously, he had always voted Labour or Lib Dem as a matter of principle. His parents never discussed politics within his earshot, but he discovered, after subtle suggestions and a few leading questions, that his mother always voted Conservative, and his father always Labour. True to their stereotypes, his mother always saved her money whilst his father always spent his. He once heard it said that the average young person (at least in Matthew's day) starts off full of idealism and radicalism when he first gets the vote, but inevitably ends up becoming an old reactionary once he experiences the reality of the world order.

Had he lost the ability to engage in left-brain thinking all of a sudden? Perhaps his left cerebral hemisphere had become exhausted through over-analytical thinking over the years? Maybe it was time for the right brain to pull its weight.
"I never knew you were left-handed," remarked Sean, the saxophonist, one evening, when they were having their customary post-practice drink. Matthew was surprised to find himself lifting the Guinness to his mouth with his left hand: he had not deliberately chosen to do so.
"I think, everything's just swapped round, I found myself trying to write with my left hand, the other day. They say you know when the right brain's

taking over, because you start to react more instinctively – gut reactions, if you like. It's been quite liberating, really, because now I no longer have to agonise over decision-making: it's a case of here's what I'm going to do and I'll apologise later in the unlikely event that I was wrong."
"Any other differences?" asked Sean.
"Well, my thought processes just seem to be dominated by vivid images. In fact - I have to tell you this - I have no desire to resume my job as a linguist."
"Why don't you come and do some music with me," suggested Sean, "and we could throw in some digital photography, too, if you like."
"I'll give it a go, I've always wanted to do something creative, and that would obviously tie in with right brain activity."

To make way for new activities, you are sometimes obliged to jettison some of old; but Matthew did not like parting with anything. It was, however, his changed view of the world that set him out on various campaigns to improve the environment that he lived in.

## Chapter forty-nine – the re-cyclist

**"At the recycling centre,**
**there are receptacles for clear bottles,**
**brown bottles and green bottles:**
**Why are there no receptacles for blue bottles?"**

**"Because there's no fly-tipping allowed!"**

Matthew liked the way deleted computer files were sent first for recycling, just in case you changed your mind about their relative importance at a later date. In non-cyber world, you could not retrieve information you had discarded and this probably explained why Matthew became a hoarder, and not a de-clutterer.

Matthew was frustrated by guarantees on products for only one year with the clear warning to anyone foolhardy enough to want to repair them that they had 'no user-serviceable parts'. How often had he gone to repair some electrical device, only to find that some killjoy had assembled it using strange triangular screws that no tool in his kit could possibly extract.

However, after a couple of unsuccessful attempts to repair mangled videotapes, he was beginning to learn how they were assembled, and could eventually fix them quite quickly. Of course you inevitably lost some of the picture and sound along the crumpled section, but it was usually only a matter of a couple of seconds. He patiently removed the small metal pillars and springs, noting their positions and how the tape meandered first to the left, then to the right, snaking its way around the plastic cartridge. It was with great satisfaction that he returned the rescued video to its delighted recipient who would otherwise have had to purchase an expensive replacement training video.

We remember how his prudent servicing of the washing-machine had given it a ten year life-span, but he was also determined not to buy a new lawn-mower when it was only the blades that had become blunt. He went to all the suppliers, including the shop that had sold him the machine five years earlier, but no one now stocked or could get hold of the part. In due course, he talked to a garage mechanic who had a number of spare parts left over from the time when they sold garden equipment.
"This is the closest match we have," explained the mechanic, "It's a couple of inches shorter than the original." Matthew took it anyway, and attached it to his lawn-mower. "There you are," he said to Anita, "It makes a perfect cut, but you just need to remember to keep the stripes ten inches wide, rather than twelve."

Anita's patience had already been tried with the repair of their alarm clock. Ever since she had attempted to vary the hour at which they were to awaken, the clock had been going off three-and-a-quarter hours too early.
"No problem," said Matthew, putting on his thinking cap, "all we need to do is change the time." He set back the time by the appropriate number of hours, and, lo and behold, the alarm started going off at the right time. British Summer Time was a bit of a challenge, but he finally worked that out, too.
"Why don't we just get a new one?" asked Anita.
"It's got sentimental value," replied Matthew, "look, here in small letters, 'made in GDR'. Most of these ended up being used to detonate bombs – this one survived."

"You're not telling me that its provenance is suspicious, are you?" asked Anita.
"It would have made a nice story that linked up with my time in East Germany, but, no, actually it belonged to my father. I know it's just a tatty lump of plastic, but I feel somehow attached to it, you know, like ***animism***?"

In town, the following day, Anita thought she had found the answer to Matthew's dilemma about whether to keep various items or throw them away.
"I've bought you a book on Feng Shui", said Anita.
"That's very kind of you", said Matthew, "what's it about?"
"Apparently, the basic idea is about allowing energy forces to flow freely through your home. If you've got a lot of useless clutter in your house, the energy gets blocked."
"Sounds moderately interesting", said Matthew and went off to digest its contents.

Anita was a martyr when it came to putting up with Matthew's regular eccentricities. It was probably only her extreme patience and concern for his welfare that stopped him paying a much earlier visit to the psychiatrist. Family life appears to normalise what would objectively be seen as clearly aberrant behaviour. Long-suffering wives often make enormous sacrifices to accommodate their somewhat disturbed husbands.

"Well?" enquired Anita, "has it convinced you that you need to get rid of all that junk you keep up in the loft?"
"Not exactly", replied Matthew, "that's all ***out-of-sight*, *out-of-mind*** stuff. What we really need to tackle, according to this book, is where we locate things downstairs, too."
"But I like the way the furniture's organised," protested Anita "How drastic are the changes you are suggesting?"

"It's more about not having things in the wrong place. Take the downstairs toilet, for example."
"What a bizarre place to start! – but go on, I am willing to be convinced."
"Apparently, mirrors amplify whatever is in proximity to them, so, if you want to be rich, for instance, you should place a mirror where it reflects symbols of wealth."
"So, what's that got to do with the toilet?" asked Anita.
"Well, that large mirror that we never got round to hanging is still propped up against the wall in the toilet and consequently it is bringing a profusion of crap into our lives!" replied Matthew.
"Take it down to the dump, then", suggested Anita.
"Job done", confirmed Matthew, ready for his next diplomatically inserted idea. "And one more thing: we've got too many empty vessels around the house; we need to put some coins in them."

Anita paused for a while, wondering what hare-brained scheme he would come up with next, and rather regretting her decision to buy the feng shui book in the first place. What she had intended as a catalyst for the disposal of worthless assets was threatening her carefully selected collection and arrangement of cherished possessions. She need not have worried. He soon became bored with this particular fad. In later years, however, he was to return to the basic concept, wondering if it could be applied psychologically. Did the arch-communicator Matthew, who was suffering from information-overload, need feng shui for the brain, perhaps?

Anita had been looking at holiday destinations, and expressed her desire to go to Morocco, Marrakech in particular. Matthew very much warmed to the idea himself and the experience was truly life-changing for both of them. In the ***souk***, they marvelled at the artisans' abilities to turn an old lamp into a teapot and vice versa, using only their hands and a small hammer. Nothing was thrown away: everything seemed to get recycled. Matthew was amazed to see ancient Peugeot cars being driven around and enquired where they had all come from originally.
"Some are from France, of course, but there a quite a few from Britain," said Abdul, the guide.
"How do they get them over here and how can it be worth it to transport second-hand vehicles so far?"
"I believe you have something called an MOT in Britain?" said Abdul.
"Yes," confirmed Matthew, "but what's that got to do with it?"
"The MOT failures are shipped to Morocco, and then we fix them and drive them for another ten years, or more." The guide suggested he check out his answer once he returned to the UK with a contact in a breaker's yard in the south of England.
"Just shows what an absolute nonsense the car scrappage scheme is, doesn't it?" said Matthew to Anita.

"Next stop Cuba," said Matthew, and Anita agreed, as it was a place she had been longing to visit, too. Necessity is the mother of invention, goes the saying, and Cuba epitomises that idea in so many ways. After travelling in a 1950's American gas-guzzler for a couple of miles, they were both high on the kerosene, or whatever other substitute fuel was being used, and could now see why we all need to be more frugal in our consumption of petrol, but they were charmed by that flashback to what was in many ways a simpler life. The car parts for the Chevrolets were unobtainable from America because of the embargo on trade the US had imposed; in any case, most of the parts would by now have become obsolete. Cubans had inherited these cars from their fathers and grandfathers and they cannibalised other vehicles, or otherwise simply made the relevant parts themselves. Even the likes of brake fluid were a strange concoction, allegedly made from household cleansers, and the like.

In Cuba, every square inch of fertile soil is devoted to growing vegetables, and, ironically, the rest of the world is having to learn from Cuba's organic way of farming. Fertilisers have been an unnecessary luxury. Matthew saw no evidence of house-building in Cuba, and asked the guide why.
"Put it this way," said Leonard, "a bag of cement costs the equivalent of three months wages. Does that answer your question? As a consequence, three generations have to live in the same house." Leonard arranged a visit so that Matthew could get a picture of local life in the country areas.

The dwelling was made of wood, with a tin roof to catch the rain-water for household use. Each family in the house had one room, with only curtains to separate the rooms and offer some privacy.
"But you all seem to like life under Fidel Castro, despite these hardships, do you honestly prefer it to the attractions of the USA?" asked Matthew.
"Put it this way, we have no guns, no drugs, no gambling and no Macdonald's, which would you choose?" Matthew thought a while, and then started to question Leonard's assertion.
"No drugs?" he queried. Leonard explained the consequences of being caught in possession of drugs: life imprisonment.
"No weapons?" asked Matthew.
"You might get the odd misuse of a machete, after the locals have had too much to drink," replied Leonard.
"Are there really no burger bars?"
"Only the one in Guantanamo Bay," replied Leonard, with a wry smile, "And all gambling is illegal – apart from dominos." Matthew recalled that, prior to Fidel's revolution, the mafia had been hoping to turn Havana into another Las Vegas.
---
It seems amazing that Matthew could recall whole paragraphs of dialogue, some of them from half a century ago. More recent conversations had become harder to remember, but perhaps that was just an inevitable

consequence of the ageing process – or maybe his brain needed some ***feng shui*** de-cluttering after all this time.

## Chapter fifty – the declutterer

Just as ***astrology*** diminished in stature as ***astronomy*** became the serious scientific subject, so ***ecology*** has experienced a similar disdain from economists with vested interests in keeping the exploitation of the Earth's resources going. Whilst it may be true that the planet goes through various cycles which have, in the past, led to reversal in the Earth's polarity, global warming, and the Ice Age, there is little doubt that mankind, as a species, is either causing, or at the very least exacerbating climate change.

So, what has ecology to do with the defragmentation process that Matthew underwent, you may wonder? Ecology has a great deal to do with how we dispose of crap. Matthew had been a rather late convert to recycling, encouraged, like many in his generation, by his own children who reprimanded him about the amount of trash he casually consigned to the dustbin. In Germany, he became a reluctant convert to renewable sources of energy, long before the UK had shown an interest: solar power, geothermal, wind and wave power, etc.

Feng Shui may have been a passing fad for some, but it taught Matthew a simple truth: you cannot be effective in life when you are surrounded by clutter. It was a hard lesson to learn, because he liked the mess that was his office. Applying the same lesson to his brain was even more effective. Clearing out all the unnecessary emotional baggage seemed to create space for new ideas and projects. On the environmental front, he imagined encouraging initiatives to re-establish sustainable forests that would help the planet return to its correct balance with clean soil, air and water. Similarly, his brain could thrive on all the nutrients supplied by his change in diet – fish oils were the most important ingredient in this – and his new exercise routine helped to maintain his positive spirit. He abandoned cerebral thinking and adopted something far more visceral – he started thinking with his gut.

Right-brain thinking produces instant results. There is no delayed gratification, like one experiences during purely left-brain thinking. The whole process became more intuitive as Matthew started to realise that he could often arrive at a better, and more immediate, decision this way. Indulging his senses, and not just the five we normally speak of, Matthew enjoyed his powers of synaesthesia that had clearly remained dormant for most of his life. Almost simultaneously, he discovered a hidden repository for his thoughts in different parts of his body: muscle memory; more precisely, emotional muscle memory.

"You say you have mixed emotions about having had to stop work, temporarily. Tell me, do you experience all of these simultaneously?" asked Sue. Matthew had to think carefully before he could answer this question.
"To be honest, I think it swings from one extreme to the other. Sometimes, I'm over the moon about not having to turn up for work on a daily basis, but then I have to admit that I miss the camaraderie." Then Sue pointed out an interesting fact,
"Your brain can handle only one emotion at a time. It's up to you to take over and tell it what you want that emotion to be, because your brain doesn't have any vested interest here. If you fail to take control and allow your early memories to set the tone, it's more likely you'll enter into a depressed state, because you'll tend to hang on to vivid memories of bad experiences and forget the good ones. If you dictate a positive tone, the optimism will prevail. And another thing; don't dwell on the connotations your brain drags up. If you do, you're straight into a negative spiral of despair; whereas if you move on to new thoughts, the traumatic experiences of your childhood will fade into insignificance."

"But I've found in some ways that pain ***is*** good for me," said Matthew. "It reminds me that I am alive. It seems to help in the learning process too." Sue endorsed this latter view,
"If learning is concomitant with embarrassment, or trauma, it is likely to be a most effective form of learning and practically impossible to erase from your memory. Remember: no pain, no gain. And as for new things, what you need to bear in mind is that information has a shelf-life. If you don't process and file it within a week, it's lost for good." Matthew got rather worried about his psychological pending tray,
"Oops!" he said. But Sue suggested a solution:
"Try to give it an emotional connotation."

Matthew was surprised,
"I thought you said I was to jettison all that emotional baggage? What's the use in cluttering up my brain with a new lot?" Sue explained.
"This time, ***you*** determine the emotion. It's probably best to make humorous connections to start with."
"Can I replace negative connotations with positive ones, too?" asked Matthew. "Well," said Sue, "I'll give you an example. You know how you cannot get a negative image of a person out of your head whenever you see him or her because he/she has hurt you emotionally and you feel powerless to retaliate and set the record straight?" Matthew nodded. "Try turning him or her into a caricature, and above all, stop thinking of the person by name: choose a ridiculously apposite nickname instead. Names are very powerful: don't allow them to have power over you."

"There's something rather disturbing about this whole process," said Matthew. "In disempowering people whom I previously perceived as

having power over me, I am reducing them to mere cardboard cut-outs. Whatever next? Will the next step be to erase them entirely from my memory?" Sue tried to reassure Matthew,
"Remember how we try never to speak ill of the dead? Once you have used your imagination to turn the bullies into ***Looney Toons,*** try to have some compassion for them by acknowledging their saving graces. Then, when you do recall their images in the dim and distant future, it will be as fond memories."

"Did you watch much TV in hospital?" asked Sue.
"Funny you should ask," said Matthew. "I couldn't stand to watch the news or any of the exciting dramas that would have been my favourite programmes before my breakdown." Sue was curious,
"So what did you choose to watch?" she enquired.
"Innocuous drivel, mostly," replied Matthew, "Soaps and Quiz Shows - that sort of thing." Sue suggested he turn over a new leaf and restrict his viewing habits, so that he could control the amount of salacious trivia bombarding his subconscious mind. "Remember," said Sue, "Your eyes are precious: treat them with respect!" Matthew was about to pass on Sue's advice to his good friend, Steve.

Steve was a genuine soul. What you saw was what you got: he was a laugh-a-minute; he provided perceptive insights into human nature; he was an accomplished jazz trumpeter and, on top of all this, he was a shrewd accountant. Given his cheeky demeanour and repartee, you might have been forgiven for assuming that his respect for institutions would be limited; but when it came to supporting his local church, Steve was a stalwart. He was generous to a fault, and his presence at Matthew's parties was an indispensible ingredient in entertaining the guests.

## Chapter fifty-one – the keen observer

***Q: How do you tune into the new ADHD channel?***
***A: You have to press the hyperactive button on your handset!***

(Jokes based on psychiatric conditions are not really PC nowadays; but they do serve a useful function in providing some light relief ***within*** the psychiatric community).

"The only saving grace for a gun is that you can use it to respond to the crap you have to endure on television," said Matthew.
"You mean like Elvis did?" said Steve, "I suppose they didn't have remote handsets in his day."
"But throwing a switch, either remotely or by getting up off your big fat arse and walking over to the television just doesn't give you the same satisfaction, does it?" said Matthew.
"I wouldn't know," said Steve, "I've only ever shot photographs."
"But surely you must agree, as a mathematician, that nowadays television is all aimed at pleasing what they so delightfully refer to as the ***lowest common denominator***."

Steve agreed about the parlous state of broadcasting,
"It ***is*** dire. So many choices of channel and yet, paradoxically, no choice at all."
"But you watch that drivel, don't you?" said Matthew, "It's like voting for politicians: it only encourages them!" Steve protested:
"I'm quite eclectic in my viewing habits, you know. I refuse to watch the salacious ones." Matthew sighed,
"Trouble is, they're all a bit like that, aren't they?"
"How do you mean?" asked Steve.
"LCD means entertainment. Entertainment equals titillation," said Matthew.

"You could try writing to ***Points of View***," said Steve, "or one of the other feedback programmes. You could even send an email." Matthew shook his head,
"It wouldn't make a blind bit of difference." Steve recalled a campaign that Matthew had contributed to,
"Didn't you once write to the Advertising Standards Authority?" Matthew recalled the response,
"I think our concerted action did have a limited effect, but the same company were soon back to their old ways, making fun of people that 'hear voices': catchy marketing idea, you see." Steve thought this through,
"So if there were concerted action, as you put it, amongst the licence payers, it might force the BBC to change our televisual diet?" Matthew again shook his head,

"that one weapon the public has is denied them."
"How do you mean?" asked Steve.
"It's illegal to refuse to pay the licence fee," said Matthew. "You have to switch the TV off instead. People must stop exposing themselves to crap, if they want to have any hope of not being brainwashed by it. Just remember: crap sticks. It doesn't matter whether it's real crap that you take on board by a process of osmosis in the real world, or artificial crap that you absorb subliminally by surrendering your powers of imagination to the fantasy industry."

"And what about reality TV?" asked Steve, thinking he'd found a crack in Matthew's argument.
"Now there's an oxymoron, if ever I've heard one," said Matthew. "You only ever get edited highlights, and most of them either staged by the production team or exaggerated by the participants. If you were watching a real life situation, it would be far too boring to bear. Like watching paint dry." Steve smiled,
"I think they've actually got programmes for ***aficionados of desiccating decoration*** on specialist channels."
"Pay-per-view?" asked Matthew.
"No," said Steve, "wallpaper's just for screen-savers." Here begins the ***punathon***.

Matthew asked Steve to close his eyes.
"What do you see?" he asked.
"What am I supposed to see?" asked Steve.
"That's exactly the response I was expecting," said Matthew. "Television conditions us all to anticipate a limited series of images. It stops us using our imagination. It's as if we've turned our own private toilets into public conveniences. Just imagine how you would feel if that actually happened. Every day having to clean up after folk with no interest in clearing up after themselves." Steve pulled a face.
"Like an episode of ***the crapped-on factor***!" he suggested.
"Do you see how this unadulterated trash can pollute your mind?" asked Matthew. "Yes," said Steve, "I see what you mean." Matthew started to analyse their choice of words.
"***Seeing*** is understanding. We should stop ***watching*** and start ***looking***. Passive watching is potentially just as damaging to your health as passive smoking." Steve needed clarification.
"What's the difference between watching and looking? They both sound like active pursuits to me."

Matthew tried to draw a direct analogy.
"The eye was the inspiration for the camera, as we all know; but subsequent inventions, like the projector, have enabled us to reverse the process. How many of us use our eyes like that?" Steve was puzzled.

"How can you project an image with your eyes?" he asked.
"There are several ways, some slightly more fanciful than others," said Matthew. "Give me the fanciful ones first," said Steve.

"You realise, Steve, that under hypnosis, both positive and negative hallucinations can be induced?" said Matthew.
"Yes, I've seen stage hypnotists convince susceptible victims either that a person is sitting in what to the audience is clearly an empty chair, or, conversely, failing to see a person who is clearly present," said Steve, "but surely that's all happening inside the victim's head?" Matthew wanted to at least sow the seeds of uncertainty in the mind of Steve, who was clearly very sceptical of the whole process.
"Steve," he said, "do you see that bright red light over there? Indulge me just for a couple of seconds, would you, please? Look at the light for a couple of seconds, then close your eyes and look over at the blank wall to your left. Now tell me what you see."

Steve acknowledged that the light reappeared on the blank wall, but added, "They're only after-images, Matthew, and in any case, the phantom light is green, which proves it's not a projection." Matthew was happy to leave this little game.
"Do you want to know how projection works?" Steve smiled,
"You mean projection of the Freudian kind, where you project your own shortcomings onto others, I assume?" Matthew responded,
"No. Though that is an interesting use of 'projection', it's not the notion I was thinking of. Perhaps you need to think of some of the major projects you have been involved with."

Steve selected an architectural project in which he had been involved, from the start, on the planning process. Matthew asked him to consider what the first stage in the project was, before any work could be done on it.
"I suppose the drawings?" he suggested.
"But even before the architect can start the drawings, what does he need to have? I'll give you a clue: it's what we've been discussing." Steve realised what Matthew was getting at,
"Oh, of course, why didn't I think of it straightaway? You mean a ***vision***." Matthew smiled.
"Precisely," he said. "Why else would we call our idea a project? People need to realise that they too, like the architect, can have a vision without being labelled a fantasist."
"So how might ordinary people reclaim control over what they see?" asked Steve.

"They could start by purchasing a video-camera and making their own films," said Matthew. "You cannot believe how empowering that can be for folk who've only ever been on the receiving end of television. They finally

feel what it is like to take control of the camera, ***looking***, instead of watching. Once they've experienced that power, they will forever scrutinise what's going on in the world with different eyes." Steve agreed,
"Yes, I can see how being the cameraman can enfranchise the man-in-the-street. It gives him authority." Matthew picked up on the latter idea,
"It's like being the author: the ***creator***, if you like." Steve took this one stage further. "You think it's like playing God?" Matthew agreed,
"Surely it's better to emulate God, than to allow yourself to be manipulated by the devil?"

Steve believed himself to be sufficiently astute, and pious, for that matter, not to be influenced in this way,
"I never allow myself to be brainwashed by television; nor the newspapers, for that matter. I'm eclectic when it comes to filtering the news."
"I don't doubt that," said Matthew, "but do you ever read foreign newspapers or watch any one of a myriad of foreign news channels?" Steve had to admit he did not, mainly because he did not want to be bothered by the idiomatic conundrums of foreign languages. Matthew dismissed this objection,
"you could watch programmes from America, Russia, India and China which are all available in English. Even though each channel will have its own hidden agenda, the very fact that you can contrast what you're hearing here with what foreign news channels are saying gives you a better insight into the 'truth'. Our far-too-parochial news blinds us to the events of greater significance happening on the other side of the globe."

"I suppose I could experiment with ***remote viewing***" said Steve, seeking to provoke Matthew into one of his frequent ventures into the paranormal.
"Don't knock it till you've tried it," said Matthew, "with a little patience, and maybe extended imagination / projection, you might be able to tap into remote locations."
"And do you just vampire-tap into GPS systems, like satnav?" said Steve.
"Who knows?" said Matthew. "All this technology might be helping us to rediscover powers we used to employ, before cultural sophistication brought with it Pyrrhonistic scepticism."

"Perhaps it's like astral projection," said Steve. "They say your soul can leave your body and go on intergalactic journeys." Matthew thought there might be something in this idea,
"Some folks recall leaving their physical bodies in near-death experiences on the operating tables in hospitals; like them, celestial dreamers can recall a bird's eye view of the room, often describing objects on the tops of cupboards that would normally remain out of sight to anyone standing in the room."

"I always go back to song lyrics for inspiration," said Matthew. "Remember the song, ***I left my heart in San Francisco***?"
"Of course," said Steve, "Tony Bennett number."
"Well," said Matthew, "Just think about that title for a moment. Could it be that when your soul fragments, certain shreds of evidence of your stay can be detected in sundry locations that you have visited or lived in around the world?"
"I see your point," said Steve, "like explorers, who left their mark on faraway lands?" "Yes," said Matthew, "or like an architect who might have bequeathed morsels of his soul to future generations in the edifices he designed." Steve added another example, "I'm sure Mozart's soul is resurrected every time we hear his music." Matthew added further examples,
"Writers, artists, generals, kings – they all leave something of themselves behind, something immortal for posterity to continue to enjoy, long after their deaths."

Steve considered the heritage of ordinary people,
"Whether it's photographs, family heirlooms or letters, everyone can leave a part of their soul behind."
"Unfortunately," said Matthew, "nobody appreciates these bequests today. 'Flog it!' seems to be the universal recommendation to families, and now that email has all but replaced letter-writing, there will be soon be no records of personal communications for future generations to peruse."
"And yet, the internet has helped folk trace their genealogy," said Steve. "It's ironic, really, that just at the time people are showing an interest in their forefathers, they're failing to leave records of their own existence for the benefit of future generations." Matthew agreed,
"Facebook, You Tube, Twitter: they'll all disappear without trace once the provider pulls the plug."

Having decided to protect his eyes from now on, Matthew next decided to focus on protection for his ears. In order to find the appropriate voice-filter, he decided to consult an expert: another friend, Carol.

To picture Carol, one need look no further than Dame Edna:
"Spooky, darling – spooky!" she would say, in close parody of Barry Humphries. Her wardrobe was, shall we say, somewhat esoteric; but the combinations of textures and colours matched her personality to a tee. The dedication she showed to the practically lost causes of the waifs and strays that consulted her to sort out their problems was commendable.

## Chapter fifty-two – the acute listener

Matthew had once been asked to shave off his beard by the ***disability police***, because it was seriously inhibiting one deaf student's ability to lip read during his lessons. He had sported a full beard for thirty years, ever since his time as a student, and he was not about to allow his own human rights to be undermined in this way. Strangely enough, once he had come out the other end of his mental breakdown, relatively unscathed, he no longer wished to keep his beard and promptly shaved it off. Since he simultaneously stopped wearing glasses, his appearance was quite drastically changed. And the medication had helped him gain two stones in weight, so that added to the new identity which he resolved to embrace. He determined not to return to his hyper-analytical former self, and indulged his creative side instead, making his ***alter ego*** complete.

Carol could not hear very well, but actually, this made her an ***acute*** listener. Like many people with a sensory impairment, she often had to encourage her other senses to overcompensate for the deficiency.
"Look at me when I'm talking to you!" Matthew's mother used to say, frustrated at his reluctance to maintain eye-contact when he was being castigated for some minor misdemeanour. In Carol's case, it was slightly different. She was inclined to say, "Look at me when you're talking to ***me***!" Matthew knew how experts in body language interpreted his rather shifty gaze, but on watching a video playback of a television interview he once gave, he observed how he always looked away just after being asked a question, and he further realised that he would invariably look away to the left when asked to recall past events and to the right, where his future intentions were being explored by the interviewer.

"It puts me off, when I try to answer a question looking someone straight in the eye," said Matthew, "it seems to interrupt the flow of my answer." Carol took hold of his face - quite a disconcerting experience the first time it happened - but he got used to it, over time. "It's like when the music teacher has to intervene manually to ensure I am adopting the right position for playing," said Matthew.
"That must make it hard to teach any subjects where physical contact is practically essential," said Carol. Matthew concurred,
"nobody dares get anywhere near kids nowadays, for obvious reasons. By the way, Carol, did you hear the one about the schools inspector who walked into a biology lesson only to find the teacher doing a striptease act?"
Carol knew some dire pun was about to surface but went along with the joke anyway,
"Go on, Matthew, what did the inspector say?" Matthew responded,
"Ms Jones, that's not what we mean by an 'enhanced disclosure'!

Carol hated the way Matthew was always keen to repeat his jokes for her benefit to ensure they had been fully understood, and she imagined other people would find this habit immensely irritating.
"It's one thing we folk with a hearing impairment often miss out on, humour, because it's often an integral aspect of the joke that the punch-line is delivered quickly. Now, I like humour in its many forms, so, in order not to miss out on my fair share, I usually select the text option when watching comedies on TV. Have you ever tried the text option, Matthew?"

Matthew used to watch English sitcoms in Germany, where the programmes were frequently dubbed, unfortunately by a limited number of actors' voices. Only Manuel in ***Faulty Towers*** seemed believable as a character, probably because Andrew Sachs had personally dubbed the part: the other familiar voices reminded the audience of roles the speakers had dubbed in programmes like Colombo, Ironside or Cannon. Matthew did, however, occasionally choose the text option:
"Where I have selected it, it's certainly been a help in following foreign films, but it's not always quite accurate, is it, Carol?" Carol agreed, but acknowledged that the facility had been a major assistance in recent years.

"Do you use texting much on your mobile phone, Carol?" asked Matthew.
"It's useful sometimes, I suppose," replied Carol.
"And e-mail, message boards and the like?" asked Matthew.
"I must admit that some of the new technological developments have really empowered people with various disabilities, but it's all very impersonal, isn't it? Imaginary friends, and all that." Matthew tried to imagine what it would be like to have a disability, but he realised that exercises where you are led around blindfolded, or fed white noise to simulate deafness, for example, go nowhere near the experience of either disability.
"After all," he said to Carol, "I know that, unlike you, I can resume my normal levels of sensory perception whenever I choose."

Carol emphasised the point,
"imagine being permanently condemned to sensory deprivation. Think what it's like for those poor bastards in Guantanamo, being subjected to torture of that kind, and you'll maybe appreciate the degree of isolation it engenders. A black bag over your head to shut out all light. People can almost imagine what it would be like to be blind; but permanent deafness – not wishing to underestimate the impact of blindness, you understand – is far worse than that."

"I don't think I can truly appreciate what you have had to cope with," said Matthew. He waited a while before asking his next question, because he wondered how Carol would take it. "Carol," he said, "do you mind if I ask you a question?" Carol was apprehensive,

"What kind of question?" she asked, sensing his hesitation in coming straight to the point. Matthew set the scene.
"You know how the likes of me are said to hear voices?" Carol nodded, realising that this was a ruse on his part, since it betokened a degree of self-disclosure.
"I think I can anticipate what you are about to ask me: you want to know if I hear voices?" Matthew shook his head.
"No, not in that 'inner conflict' kind of way. I was curious to know whether you can replay conversations in your head." Carol smiled.
"You mean to compensate for the conversations I can no longer hear?"

Matthew tried to explain,
"When I'm writing, it's like a whole series of conversations between the characters emerging. I can hear them all making jokes, arguing their points, shouting each other down, at times. How about you?" Carol agreed,
"The characters really come to life. You almost want to hug them, they seem so real." Matthew continued,
"And do they speak quietly or at a normal level?" Carol smiled somewhat condescendingly,
"depends what you mean by ***normal.***" Matthew was not put off,
"does the ***volume*** of their individual speeches vary?"

Carol decided to reverse roles with Matthew, just to put an end to his incessant interrogation mode,
"When you, with your psychiatric condition, hear voices, are they whispering to you or shouting at you?" Matthew had to think for a while about his answer to this unexpected question.
"When I'm paranoid, I suppose it's like an array of whispering tormentors, bullying me into self-destructive actions, or at least self-critical sentiments that lead to apparent clumsiness or sometimes to major cock-ups. When they do finally precipitate the inevitable disaster on my part, it's the louder voices that take over, burying me in a storm of profanities in response to my ineptitude." Carol chose to reciprocate, now that Matthew had described a half-way comparable experience,
"Yes, the volume does vary," she said, "but you might have to check with Les about the technicalities of what I actually hear."

Les was a sound engineer with a keen ear for balanced sound and an excellent grasp of how acoustics worked.
"A bit grainy," said Les.
"Pardon," said Matthew, "I don't understand." Les put it in terms he knew Matthew would appreciate,
"Carol is experiencing a veritable cacophony of sound. You know how you've got your musical ***left*** ear, sending sounds off to your right cerebral hemisphere, so you stick your finger in your right ear to block off all the

distorted noise?" Matthew nodded, and observed that he also had a preferred telephone ear, his right ear,
"so my right ear's for speech, I take it?"
"Possibly," said Les, "though you'll probably find you put the receiver to whichever side is most convenient at the time, particularly if you need your right hand to write down details."

"Les, have you heard of that phenomenon called the ***cocktail party syndrome***?" asked Matthew.
"Where you can allegedly zero in on conversations further away?" asked Les.
"Yes," said Matthew, "only sometimes I find my ears taking on a life of their own. There's a conversation going on right next to me, but I either can't follow it, or I miss key parts of it, because background conversations are coming through more clearly." Carol rejoined the conversation,
"Matthew," she said, "I think you should get your hearing checked out, just to be on the safe side."

Matthew protested,
"There's nothing wrong with my hearing, as far as I know; it's probably just my inability to concentrate for longer periods. Also, it's that mimicry thing: my ears filter out normal voices and select only interesting ones." Carol frowned,
"Are you saying we're too boring to listen to?" she asked.
"No, it's not that at all," said Matthew, "it's got more to do with the way certain people speak. If they articulate the words well, modulate the frequency of their voices, speak clearly, concisely and with emphasis on certain syllables, my ears are naturally more attracted to those sounds than to the hurriedly expressed mumblings emanating from a colleague in a neighbouring seat."

Carol recalled a line from an old Cilla Black song, ***Sing a Rainbow***,
"Listen with your eyes, listen with your eyes..." she said, "you know, Matthew, I really miss the kaleidoscope of sound that I was fortunate enough to experience when I was a child. At least, I have the memories of what I could perceive then. Hearing aids are okay under certain circumstances, but they really don't help when you're trying to listen to noisy music in a pub. It's just an unpleasant din. I prefer not to go out. Preferring to stay at home now, in your own immortal words – or was it those of REM[28]? - I'm receptive only to ***the very rarest of frequencies***."

---

[28] The band, REM, recorded ***Rare Frequencies***

## Chapter fifty-three – the joker

One very irritating habit, commonly shared by bi polar sufferers is the uncontrollable desire to indulge in what is referred to as 'manic punning'. Throughout their conversations with you, they are on the look-out for plays on words. There is the occasional gem amongst these, but you have to put up with a whole torrent of nonsense before one turns up.

Matthew developed the ability to recall not only the joke, but also the comedian who told it and the precise time and place of its first airing. He liked one-liners such as the Les Dawson joke about the man who was forced to spent a freezing cold winter's night out in the vegetable patch, and woke up 'frozen to the marrow'.

One joke remained with him from his teenage years:

***A man travels back in time to the Stone Age and observes a man and woman rubbing two sticks together.***
***"What are you doing?" he asks, curious about the purpose of such activity.***
***"We're making love," came the reply.***
***"God, that's not much fun, is it?" said the man.***
***"You should see how we make fire!" replied the couple.***

He remembered David Frost telling the joke about the Latin student whose marriage was annulled because when asked to conjugate, he declined.

He could even go back to the humour around in his father's day in recalling the work of Sandy Powell. The latter's sketches used to be recorded on the old gramophone records, some of which were still in Matthew's possession. Of course, the family had parted with the old machine long ago, but he remembered how frequently the needles had to be changed before the diamond stylus came along. Like Matthew, Sandy played several roles. At one point, he was Sandy the tram-conductor; at another, he was Sandy, the radio ham. The jokes were pretty naf:

***The soles on my shoes were so thin, if I stood on a halfpenny, I could tell you if it was heads or tails!***

Matthew once bought a book of cartoons which identified four basic categories of humour – sex, violence, intellectual jokes and nonsense jokes. According to your personality, it was said, you would tend to gravitate towards comedians that matched your preference. Matthew found that he tended to prefer satire and intellectual humour and selected the corresponding TV programmes. He did not much appreciate the crass sexual jokes or the ones deriving pleasure from violence, but he went along with them where a clever twist was added to them: Peter's joke, for example, where the woman went into a bar asking for a ***double entendre***, and the barman 'gave her one'; or Don's one about the narcissistic procrastinator who fancied himself but 'could not quite get round to it'.

Slapstick, on the other hand, did not appeal to him much. He had gone to see a pantomime at the Alhambra Theatre in Bradford with his mates. Ken Dodd had combined his usual routine with a 'Mr Pastry' interlude and a ball of dough had landed in Matthew's lap.
"Chuck it back!" shouted his mates, in chorus. Not having a good aim at the best of times, Matthew merely succeeded in hitting the drum-kit in the orchestral pit, much to the delight of the audience, if not the percussionist.

After seeing a show in Skinandis Night Club, Thurso, Matthew took it upon himself to have a chat with one of a team of stand-up comedians who were completing a tour that supported a mental health charity. Vladimir MacTavish, AKA Paul, was quite open about how frequently comedians are the very people who plunge into deep depression.
"I suppose it's inevitable, really," said Paul.
"How do you mean?" asked Matthew.
"Imagine the stress of stand-up. Either it's going really well and you've got the audience eating out of your hand, in which case your manic boost can take you into stratospheric levels of euphoria; alternatively it's going badly – through no fault of your own – and you're just not getting a reaction: not even booing or rotten tomatoes, and this sends you down into the depths of despair. Are you a performer, Matthew?"

"I've never done stand-up, but I can empathise with your situation through my experiences of playing with the jazz band," said Matthew. "Again, it can put you on a real high, when the audience are dancing and clearly enjoying the music, but – and this is irrespective of the fee paid, or the prestigious nature of the venue – if the band was there just for 'wallpaper', you can feel very flat after the event."

## Chapter fifty-four – the musician

Matthew was once the proud owner of a Gibson 335 cherry guitar which had cost him an arm and a leg in the seventies. He had used the cash from the sale of his house to buy it and was now living in a rented flat on the ninth floor of a skyscraper just outside Slough. Paradoxically, some five years later he was forced to sell the guitar to a blind musician called Lee Stirling in order to get the deposit for a house in Manchester. There is a lesson here for those who mistakenly thought that the value of property is always going up. As anyone who purchased a Fender or Gibson in their youth will have realised, such treasures are a much better investment, and not just for their financial return.

"So many folk living their lives vicariously," Matthew said to Anita, "Haven't they realized, in the words of Bob Dylan:

***You shouldn't let other people get your kicks for you.***

"I take it you've considered the possibility that this criticism might apply to yourself?" suggested Anita.
"I think I would've succeeded as a composer," said Matthew, "if I'd been single-minded about my career and not had to opt for a more secure profession."
"But you had no choice, in the circumstances," acknowledged Anita. "We'd have starved if you hadn't taken up teaching."
"That's perfectly true," acknowledged Matthew, "though I'm also thinking back to when I was just a mere fourteen-year-old and really enjoying music which had just been introduced into the grammar school. If my parents had kicked up more of a fuss at the options stage, I'm sure I'd have got to study music which was, in fact, my first choice. Unfortunately, other forces were at work which neither I, nor my parents, fully understood. As I later discovered when I myself became a teacher, true pupil choice is very restricted, and is often based on the enlightened self-interest of the teachers. Rather than ***let the market decide***, classes had been rigged to ensure the viability of established 'academic' subjects taught by masters who had spent their entire teaching-careers at the school, and these new 'Mickey Mouse' subjects, such as music (that grammar schools rarely took seriously) were the inevitable casualties."

"It's still a big issue even nowadays," said Anita. "The teachers still tend to steer pupils into careers they deem to be more appropriate for them. ***Fear of failure*** predominates today and the kids just don't get stretched at all. If they do show undue ambition, they are tactfully told to consider something less academically demanding. And, if it's not the teachers, it's the parents vicariously trying to impose their own ambitions onto their children instead of listening to them, and finding out what they actually ***want*** to do."

"I remember how hard it was for us as parents, ambitious for our son to go to Cambridge," said Matthew.
"But he had other ideas, didn't he?" said Anita.
"I suppose he'd not have put his heart into it, if he felt it wasn't his choice. Anyway, it's all turned out just fine in the end, as far as I can see."
"And what about Kate?" asked Matthew.
"Now there's an enigma," said Anita, "no apparent pressure from anyone for her to pursue any particular career, and yet she never seemed to have any obvious career in mind for herself, as I recall?"

"Do you remember how fantastically good she was at art?" asked Matthew, "I think she might have developed those skills, if she'd been given the chance."
"She's another polymath, a bit like yourself," said Anita, "It's a curse to be quite good at everything, because you're spoilt for choice, and you end up not being able to focus on one specific career."
"That's something I hadn't considered, until Burkhart pointed it out," said Matthew, "I suppose that trying to keep two, or sometimes three jobs going simultaneously often had a seriously negative impact on my promotion prospects."

"Mum always wanted to be a physician, didn't she, Dad?" said Kate, "Nursing took her part-way towards achieving her goals, and now she can be proud of the fact that she is effectively a doctor, practising alternative medicine; behoven to no vested interest group, unlike most medical practitioners. I think I too see myself as working in a caring profession: maybe I'm just following in her footsteps, at some subconscious level. I did the computing degree in an attempt to match up to my brother's achievements. I thought that might finally gain your respect."

"Maybe I was trying to compensate for not getting the breaks in Music myself, when I took you both off for piano and violin lessons," said Matthew, "You must surely appreciate being able to play so many instruments? I can still picture you playing keyboards in that heavy-metal band." Kate smiled.
"Were you secretly envious?" she enquired.
"I was then - I do have to admit that. Of course, old has-beens, or more accurately ***never-has-beens*** like myself, would have been laughed off the stage in Manchester. At least up here in the Highlands, ageism isn't so obvious, so we all get a chance to realize our ambitions, even if we're just medium-sized fish in a tiny pond."

Matthew later resolved to ask his old friend, Donnie, the sound engineer, to help him make a CD of all the songs he had written back in the sixties. A recording schedule was established so that it would take them exactly twenty-six weeks to put down thirteen tracks. Every Saturday, they would devote about eight hours to the task, first of all, laying down an appropriate drum rhythm, then Matthew would multi-track bass, guitar, keyboards and rhythm guitar, before adding the vocals, sometimes even adding a harmony. In truth, it was much harder to achieve the necessary synchronisation than he had anticipated, but he was delighted with the end-product, mainly because it fulfilled an aim he had had as a teenager. Thanks to Donnie's technical expertise, they were able, on one track, to recreate a whole orchestra of guitars with all the impact of stereo.

Music is a kind of magic, but Matthew, the Sorcerer's Apprentice, also enjoyed the power that the so-called dark arts could give to a dabbler in the occult, like himself.

## Chapter fifty-five– the magician

It was perhaps not particularly surprising, given, as we know, that one of Matthew's favourite words was ***fascinating***, that the many synonyms of this word lead us into the realms of sorcery and magic. He had read Nietzsche's ***Also sprach Zarathustra*** and discovered that the notion of the Magi, the three wise men who visited Christ, may, like Zarathustra himself, link back ultimately to the ancient civilisation of the Persians. Maybe, after a lifetime of pursuing Mazda, the unattainable light, Matthew was now ready to embrace the darker side of life. He did not have the physique to follow the dreams of Mr Apollo, as the Bonzo Dog Band advised. It was Dionysus who now beckoned, with his intoxicating ways.

Matthew once lived in a house that backed onto a church and had, as a child, detected ***strange goings on***, as his mother described them. From the Sci-Fi films he had seen, he put it all down to the activities of ***poltergeists*** in the company of disturbed adolescents, such as himself. Objects moved, light switches were heard from the church next door in the middle of the night, but nothing drastic enough happened to make his family consider moving house.

One weekend, however, when Sylvia, his girl-friend, was visiting, she and Matthew were sitting quietly around midnight, having a chat, when they both detected a sudden drop in temperature. Even Judy, the family's pet cat, clearly sensed something odd was going on, because her fur stood up on end and her normally domesticated facial features suddenly morphed into the stare of a wild-cat. Just as they were about head off to bed, the musical box, which stood on the mantel-piece, suddenly started playing Mozart's ***The Magic Flute***. This seemed inexplicable to Matthew, who knew that its clockwork mechanism had stopped working ages ago. Matthew had brought back the musical box as a souvenir of Vienna, where he and Sylvia previously met up.

Matthew later discovered Mozart's links to Masonic rituals and, of course, one of the characters in ***die Zauberflöte*** is Sarastro (Zarathustra). On two separate occasions Matthew had been invited to join the masons himself, but had refused, mainly because, like Groucho Marx, he did not want to belong to any club that would accept him as a member. He had observed a great deal of positive work the masons did for charity, but did not like the ***old school tie*** implications of such an association.

This was not to be the only occasion where Matthew's presence appeared to trigger bizarre events. In 1972, staying with friends in Highworth, Wiltshire, a town notorious for its alleged haunted pubs, Matthew had slept upstairs in a house in the High Street. In the morning, he awakened to find an abundance of white berries in a pile by his bed. Try as he may, he could not find an explanation; nor could the family whose house it was. Again, this manifestation had been accompanied by a sudden drop in temperature. Had he, however unwittingly, triggered some form of psychokinesis to produce this effect, he wondered.

---

Fast forward to the year 2001 in Thurso, Caithness.
"Just a bit of fun," said Theodora. "Do come, there'll be lots of people you know." Somewhat reluctantly, Matthew dragged himself off to the séance, armed with a pack of Tatwa cards and a crystal ball. The latter had been purchased some time before from a shop specialising in new age gifts.
"Now you realise," said Cassandra***, the prophetess ignored by men,*** "that there's no guarantee accompanying this sale, don't you?"
"No guarantee of what?" asked Matthew.
"We've had folk wanting their money back, claiming the crystal ball didn't work." Matthew smiled,
"I think it's more about having a feature to concentrate on, rather than actually conjuring up images within the sphere," he said. "I'll give you an analogy. We invented the camera to mimic the functions of the eye. We've even captured moving images. To replay the images, we have to ***project*** them onto a screen. Imagine our eyes being capable of doing the same thing. You get the idea?" Cassandra blinked and then stared at the blank wall.
"So you're saying that purely through the power of your own concentration, you can conjure up all kinds of images?"
"That's about right," said Matthew.

As a teenager, he had dabbled with Ouija boards[29] and with scrying, but, like most teenagers had quickly been frightened off by the uncanny accuracy of the predictions. He worried about summoning up demons from the abyss, in the manner of Aleister Crowley, or John Dee, the famous mathematician to Queen Elisabeth I . When he arrived at Theodora's séance, he was the only male amongst an assembly of nine delectable young ladies and initially found the experience somewhat daunting. However, he soon found his party-tricks in demand, and started off by giving graphological readings to the assembled guests. Having thus entralled the ladies, he proceeded to introduce the Tatwa cards. He knew the palmist in the room next-door would be using tarot cards to help with her own readings, so he deemed this an appropriate sideshow to the main event.

The ladies knew Matthew dabbled in numerology and quizzed him on its significance. "Well, take this young lady, for example," said Matthew, "As

---

[29] French/German for "yes"

a ***two***, her strengths lie in diplomacy. This would suggest that she functions best as a mediator, arbitrator or advocate." The young lady replied,
"In my time, I've been all three, originally as a trade union representative, but latterly, as a volunteer." Matthew continued,
"You're allegedly a spiritual idealist, but you need to be aware that you have a tendency towards intolerance of others' opinions." Theodora smiled.
"Quite accurate, in her case, then?" she confirmed.

"Time to get out the crystal ball," said Theodora, "we all want to know the future." Removing the cloth from the orb, Matthew focussed upon the glass, through not with his ***third eye*** like you sometimes can do with the Tatwa cards.
"It's a very artificial construct, you know," said Matthew, "our idea of time. Past, present and future are really all one."
"But surely," said Theodora, "only the past can impact on the present or the future, and the present on the future."
"Yes, you're partly right," said Matthew, "You'll have heard of self-fulfilling prophesies and gypsies' curses? If enough people believe something is going to happen, the ***World Will*** says it will happen. A bit like the power of prayer, in some ways. So, if we all go about saying the planet is doomed and don't do anything to rectify the problem, then that prophesy will probably come true, too."

Theodora needed to understand how the future could impact on the present.
"Think of our generation's impact on the past," said Matthew. "What is now ***reality*** existed once only in the ***imagination*** of inventors like Leonardo da Vinci. Remember, our brains can't tell the difference between reality and fantasy. Anything that can be imagined can also be realised. Perhaps we are only witnessing history repeating itself as successive civilisations reach the peak of their inventive abilities, only to be lost beneath the waves, like Atlantis, with her secrets still hiding somewhere beneath the feet of the Sphinx."

"What did you see in your crystal ball?" asked Cassandra.
"Nothing that would've gone down well at a dinner-party," said Matthew. "The fate of the ***economy*** runs hand-in-hand with the ***ecology*** of the planet. As those in charge of the financial stewardship of the Earth fail to distribute its wealth on an equitable basis, so the Earth herself decides to seek retribution for her rape and pillage, wrestling to compensate for the centuries of devastation, deforestation and pollution that mankind has caused. Her wrath will be clear from the extreme weather patterns that will inevitably face the world, and only by countries coming together, instead of fighting one another, will the Earth be saved."

Cassandra took a sharp intake of breath.

"Sounds pretty apocalyptic, if you ask me. So when's all this due to happen?" Matthew paused...
"It's fairly imminent, actually," he said, "but try coming back to me in 2012, the year of the London Olympics, if we're both still around, and we'll see if the Earth has changed polarity by then. Who knows, they might have to make it the Winter Olympics! Numerologically speaking, that year's a ***five***, and the Western World hasn't fared too well with the number five."

Cassandra sought clarification, "Give me an example!" Matthew wondered if she would put it all down to coincidence, but he gave her his best shot, "Take 9/11. If you add up the figures in the date 9/11/2001 you arrive at the number ***five.*** There were originally to have been five suicide pilots. One of the targets was the ***pent***agon, etc, etc."
"You'll be linking in some mystical connection with a ***pent***acle next," said Cassandra. "Well, don't forget the risk associated with the adventure and opportunity offered by the number five has to be kept in check by the responsibility for safety embodied by number six," said Matthew.
"Maybe it's time to put a ***hex*** on future events!" said Cassandra. The etymologist within Matthew protested
"That word comes from the Germanic word for witch, ***die Hexe*** - not the Greek for six!"

"And did you get any information relevant to you, personally?" asked Cassandra. "Well," said Matthew, "it was all very hazy, but for Luke, who is yet to be born, the sky is the limit. If he chooses to, he can circum-navigate the universe."
"Will you have other grandchildren and great-grandchildren?" asked Cassandra.
"I don't honestly know, but there will be a female relation by the name of Eleanor whom I can see making what we can presently only describe as documentary movies, though they appear to be much more elaborate affairs. Just as Luke is a sky-walker, Eleanor seems to be plumbing the depths of the oceans, looking for solutions to fix the future ecological disasters facing the Earth."

Matthew restricted his magic to pure entertainment, as he liked the way it cheered people up. Sometimes, however, he wished he could just wave a magic wand to change some of the bad ways of the world for the better.

## Chapter fifty-six – the idealist

"Nothing's ever what it claims to be, is it?" suggested Matthew to Neil, a doctor friend of his who also happened to have a personal insight into what treatment looks like from a patient's point of view.
"How do you mean?" asked Neil.
"Well, take the inappropriately named ***National Health Service***. They should be held to account under the Trades Description Act. Let's take the first misnomer. Since the decision as to what treatment you receive is based largely on a post-code lottery, the system can't claim to give equal coverage ***nationally***. Secondly, you're surely not trying to pretend that it's got anything at all to do with ***health***? Most folk would be healthier if they avoided doctors and hospitals altogether – just take ***clostridium difficile*** for starters, the hospital acquired infection. The system's more about illness than health; it's reactive rather than proactive; not about prevention at all – which brings me to my third point…"
"Wasn't that enough!" protested Neil, "We really do try our best, you know!"
"My third point is that anyone who provides a ***service*** has forgotten what the word means. It's no longer a service; it's an industry, just like the so-called 'service industry', and it relies for its profits on patients returning, just like drug-pushers rely on their addicts coming back for more. I can just imagine what my GP is thinking as she suggests I get my cholesterol checked, 'Hmm, healthy looking specimen here, let's get him to sign up to the 'worried-well' brigade. That'll help achieve our targets for this month.'

Neil smiled sardonically,
"Such cynicism! Anyway, assuming you were in government in charge of Health, what changes would ***you*** make?" Matthew had thought about this scenario before and so was able to come up with his own manifesto fairly promptly.
"For one thing, the NHS is far too bureaucratic, labyrinthine and unwieldy. For another, its relationship with the pharmaceutical industry is far too cosy. Thirdly, it's allowed itself to get privatised by the back door through allowing the gradual erosion of the State's control and handing it over piecemeal to the States: American health practices are with us already."
"Those are all things you say are wrong with the NHS," said Neil, "What would you put in its place?"

"It needs a total rethink," said Matthew. "The whole process is so wasteful. So many drugs prescribed unnecessarily, especially for mild depression. We've created a dependency culture. We encourage individuals not to take responsibility for themselves. You still get treated like a baby whenever you have dealings with a nurse – what's that all about? Baby-language abounds:

'let's get your jim-jams on now. Have we taken ***our*** medication? Doctor Rosemary says no,' etc."

"So where would you start?" asked Neil, desperately trying to imagine what Matthew had in mind.
"Use the money saved from all the iatrogenic illnesses to pay for the operations and cancer treatments that the NHS allegedly can't afford. You could save a fortune just by cutting out the enormous cost of drugs prescribed for mild depression. Instead of drugs, a little CBT in the right direction could get patients away from self-obsession, and maybe into deriving some small comfort out of helping others, for a change." "You're not very sympathetic, are you?" said Neil.
"It worked for me," said Matthew, "that's all I can say. Focussing on the issues of someone else was therapeutic for me as well as my client: it was a win/win situation." "If you ask me," said Neil, "Some folk just want to be ill. They'll do anything to get me to write a sick-note."
"Again," said Matthew, "it's part of that baby-world. They remember their mothers indulging them when they were sick children, and they subconsciously want to return to that mollycoddled existence. I'm afraid Nanny has to go, now they've grown up."

"You'll be wanting to seriously reduce benefits, too, I imagine?" said Neil.
"It's not out of spite," said Matthew. "Benefits payments are routinely supplemented by a little wheeling and dealing, not exactly legit, but if you're part of that community, you're expected to buy some dodgy goods at knockdown prices, probably nicked off your next door neighbour, otherwise you become a pariah, with all the persecution that can engender. 'I have a life-style to maintain!' claimed one guy, when I asked him why he hadn't paid his rent for six months. The notion that you can't have what you can't afford simply never occurred to him. I believe that in the current downturn in the economy, some people are in serious need of a reality check."

"Any thoughts about education?" asked Neil.
"Don't get me started!" replied Matthew. "All schools are an anachronism. They're at best like open prisons for kids, a child-minding service where the minders are so hamstrung by the regulations that the bullies can get away with murder. Let them learn at home on their computers, for God' sake."
"Only problem is," said Neil, "then, you have no training in social integration. The kids won't get any practice for the real world if they don't learn how to get along with one another."
"I think most of them get quite a shock once they realise the adult world bears little resemblance to their cotton-wool existence in schools nowadays," said Matthew.

But before he set about trying to put things right, Matthew needed the advice of Alice about how to improve the world.

## Chapter fifty-seven – the supporter

Just as he had taken an interest in fixing inanimate objects, Matthew developed a passion for trying to fix broken people. Admittedly this came about more recently after he himself had undergone a mental breakdown, but even in his teaching career, he had been as much concerned about his students' physical and mental well-being as in their academic advancement. Perhaps, he observed, it had come from his mother. As a child, he had accompanied her on her frequent visits to ageing and ailing friends and he had picked up subliminally on that notion of ***being there*** for people, regardless of what they had done or what had happened to them. ***A friend in need is a friend indeed*** ran the saying and he did his best to remain constant to his friends.

Not that he had had many close friends at school, or even at university. He had always been very much a loner, with his own individual agenda. Maybe this defiance had alienated him from his peer group. Stealing apples from the school orchard had been about the only crime he had ever committed as part of the gang, and, whether brainwashed into him by his religious upbringing, or, as he himself liked to believe, representing an attempt to adhere to his own sense of moral values, his conscience would never have allowed him to transgress, in any way.

Discovering that an acquaintance had been sentenced to a lengthy stay in a maximum security prison, Matthew resolved to pay him a visit. Again the phrase ***out-of-sight, out-of-mind*** alerted him to the convenient way criminals can be forgotten by society once they are behind bars. Matthew had never been inside a prison before and inevitably got all the prison etiquette wrong. He took along presents, most of which were confiscated or retained for collection when he subsequently departed from the prison. Entering the prison as a visitor, he soon found, was at least as invasive an experience as that to which the prisoners themselves were subjected. Strip-searches were not uncommon, bearing in mind the attempts many visitors would make to smuggle in drugs.

Arriving at the fixed furniture in an open area that constituted the meeting point, he took a seat, only to have it pointed out to him by Liam, the prisoner, that he had chosen the blue seat and not one of the orange seats reserved for guests. He kept up conversations and correspondence by mail until Liam was released. It was hard never to ask what his crime had been, but he believed that any such question would automatically have undermined their relationship because he might have been perceived to be passing judgement.

Having himself become one of the ***invisible idiots*** when he was detained for a relatively brief stay in a psychiatric hospital, Matthew knew only too well how valuable regular contact from outside can be. Barbara, his own "beautiful stranger" had established contact, even though he had hardly known her except as a passing acquaintance at work. This loyalty was something he admired in others, though he often felt he fell far short of maintaining that quality in himself: he always eventually felt the need to move on, perhaps through fear of long-term co-dependency issues.

And yet there were other friendships that seemed to prevail, despite being what others might regard as past their sell-by date. Matthew had one such friend whom he trusted above all others. Whenever he encountered what he regarded as an insurmountable problem, he knew he could share it with Alice - hopefully without overburdening her with its intricacies. Alice was a rare phenomenon nowadays – she was a person with genuine integrity who spoke up for people, even though she knew it would be no good for her own personal advancement. She had all the qualities you could have desired in a leader: she was dynamic, charismatic, caring, self-effacing, thoroughly reliable and trustworthy, politically and socially engaged; resolute, indefatigable, intuitive and an astute negotiator. In addition, she was charming, had an excellent sense of humour and would never put off listening to a friend in need, despite always having a mountain of work to deal with.

"A problem shared is a problem doubled!" he mused, thinking of all those deserving cases that he and his fellow professionals had taken on to try to represent fairly the interests of more vulnerable adults.
"Yet sometimes," said Alice, "you can't keep things to yourself, just allowing them to fester; you need someone who can give a second opinion. Often it is simply the opportunity to voice your innermost thoughts, to externalise your churning emotions, that you need. You are not necessarily looking for a solution, just for someone to spell out some possible alternatives." Matthew recognised at such moments that clearing his head was analogous with detoxing his gut,
"Much of what is stored in my brain is cerebral and therefore intellectual and philosophical; but I have to acknowledge that there is also a great deal of visceral stuff in there, ripe for major surgery."

Growing up, he had almost prided himself on keeping his emotions in check.
"I don't feel pain", he claimed one day, as he meticulously removed the head of a match, stuck it onto the middle finger-tip of his left hand, before striking it against the side of the matchbox. A flame appeared from his outstretched hand, in a vague reminiscence of an image of the devil, that he recalled from a short film he had seen as a young boy when he briefly attended the Band of Hope. The two main characters in the film were Mr

Nick O'Teen and Mr L.K. Hall. Nowadays the content would have given the film at least a 15 rating, but he and his fellow seven-year-olds were, if anything, intrigued by the experience. If the intention had been to put kids off booze and fags through a kind of aversion-therapy, the film had been a spectacular failure. From what Matthew could remember, the vast majority of that impressionable audience had gone on to become either pyromaniacs or dipsomaniacs.

Through self-hypnosis, Matthew had taught himself to reach a very high pain threshold, just in case – he reassured himself – he ever landed up in the hands of torturers. Matthew subsequently decided to see if his new-found talent for hypnosis could be used ***therapeutically*** on others. He decided to practise first on Anita, his wife. Anita had experienced severe pain from time to time and was a not-too-reluctant guinea-pig. In a spirit of trial-and-error, he developed a combination of the power of suggestion and laying-on-of-hands and succeeded in relieving her pain by a process of ***dissipation,*** as he called it. He also found that the technique worked quite well on his daughter, Kate, who suffered from recurrent migraines, though he had lingering concerns about the long-term effects of her suggestibility under hypnosis.

Sometimes he would suggest to others how to achieve this state of mind as you sat in the dentist's chair,
"You must visualise the mental image of the body, where everything close to the brain is gigantic, whilst arms and legs are perceived as minute," he said to Alice. "Imagine the pain - which you currently feel acute and localised in your upper front gum area - as a movable sensation. On the assumption that pain might be capable of being diluted by spreading it out, maybe you can effectively raise your pain-threshold by distributing it out to the far reaches of your entire body." Originally, Matthew had not fully comprehended the distinction between ***acute*** pain and ***chronic*** pain, but after a quick look in his etymological dictionary, the difference became apparent: the first related to the Latin for needle, the second to the Greek for time. Misinterpretations and mistranslations over the years had led to our rather cavalier use of the two terms. Suffice it to say, he focussed his attentions on the acute variety.

"So many damaged people out there", he said one day to Alice. "Where do I start?" It had been his firm belief that health - both physical and mental - flourishes once the person stops self-obsessing. "The 'worried well' are pivotal to the proliferation of the ***health*** industry. The whole system", he remarked, "is geared towards dependency. Whether that means dependence on drugs or dependence on other people, it stops the individual taking his own decision to recover. It's a strange contradiction that Thatcherite politics, focussing on the individual (which you might assume would make us all more self-reliant) has led to the casualties of this very philosophy desperately needing other people (whose lives and opinions they wouldn't normally give a damn about) to feel sorry for them."

Alice thought for a while, and then enquired whether he had come up with any kind of solution to this now virtually global phenomenon.
"Now I know I can't save the world. I wouldn't be so presumptuous. In any case, with my 'diagnosis', it might smack of delusions of grandeur, or messianic zeal." Alice was encouraging,
"So, come on, Matthew, you could at least make a start at the local level, what's your remedy?"
"All I can say, Alice, is that it worked for me. As soon as I started really listening to the plight of others, I realised that all my own aches and pains vanished, and my depression lifted".
"Make someone happy, and you will be happy, too", said Alice, remembering the deep satisfaction she had experienced, often after a relatively minor gesture on her part such as purchasing some flowers, when a female friend's eyes had lit up and a genuine smile had appeared on her face.

"But why do you devote so much of your precious time to so many lost causes and hopeless cases?" asked Alice.
"I can't allow myself to judge the efficacy of my involvement", replied Matthew, "I suppose it's a bit like being a solicitor, some you win, some you lose. In any case, often what seems to have been a total waste of time on the day transmogrifies into a major victory for common sense that leads eventually to positive changes in society."
"You should have been a politician", remarked Alice.

## Chapter fifty-eight – the campaigner

"It's just not right, the way the powers-that-be assume they can walk in and take over people's lives like that," said Matthew, "whatever happened to the notion that an Englishman's home is his castle?"
"It's all an illusion," said Alice, "People think that once they own property, they're somehow immune from intervention by the State, but they're profoundly wrong."

"When I was single, and living alone in rented accommodation," said Matthew, "I realised how potentially vulnerable I was. Representatives of the authorities would walk unannounced into my home and immediately start to comment unfavourably on the general untidiness of my dwelling. From the state of the - as yet - unwashed cups and plates, they decided I needed taking in hand, and when they discovered that I did not eat at normal meal-times and slept in till midday at weekends, they were just about ready to have me put into residential accommodation.
"You're what we call the ***at risk*** category," they would say, "You're male and over fifty. That means you're clearly unhealthy, lacking exercise and incapable of managing your own affairs."
"I'm only having two affairs at the moment," said Matthew, mischievously, "and the two young ladies are both quite happy with the arrangement!"
"Don't be so flippant; you know what we mean," said the social worker.

Later, in another existence, Matthew had occasion to visit the very same social worker in a ***social*** capacity and commented rather less unfavourably on her messy surroundings:
"You're obviously not suffering from obsessive compulsive disorder!" he said, pointedly.
"I know what you're getting at," said the social worker, "it's just that we spend so much time organising other people's lives, we don't get the chance to organise our own." The ***moat and beam*** hypocrisy sprang to mind.

"But surely they don't treat landed gentry like that?" asked Matthew.
"You'd be surprised," said Alice. "Folk are easily picked off if they don't have powerful friends. How frequently have you seen an ageing couple amass a little wealth for their offspring, only to find it confiscated by the powers-that-be to pay for their stay in residential accommodation. Often, they aren't even aware that their funds are being used in this way. And it helps, of course, if they are deemed to be going senile. 'Incapacity', it's called. If they fail to answer correctly the psychiatrist's set of questions, that's their soul signed, sealed and delivered. And if they're sectioned into the bargain, that's the State taking over their mind as well as their money."
"The State doesn't love its citizens, very much, does it?" said Matthew, "It only wants them for their bodies. Whatever happened to ***habeas corpus***?"

"I think you might be thinking of detention ***sine die***," said Alice.
"So they're still using Latin to keep the plebs in order: that's what the clergy used to do before we got universal education," said Matthew.

"Would you like to play a game, Alice; a game, the outcome of which could have dire consequences for you personally?" asked Matthew.
"Couldn't we just ***simulate*** the game?" asked Alice.
"Okay," said Matthew, "It's like ***twenty questions***, only in this exercise there are thirty[30]. Now, first of all, Alice, I need to assess your level of ***arousal***." This was getting quite kinky, even by Alice's standards, and she seriously felt like making a tactical exit, but Matthew reassured her, stressing that he had no hesitation in assessing her as ***alert*** as opposed to 'drowsy' or 'comatose'.

Matthew launched the first of his barrage of questions,
"What's the date today?"
"Can I consult my diary?" asked Alice.
"Certainly not," said Matthew, and I've turned the calendar round as well so you can't cheat. Second question:
"Who is the Prime Minister of the United Kingdom?" Alice smiled.
"Gordon Brown. Though by tomorrow it could well be someone else!" Matthew frowned.
"Now for the memory bit: I'm going to recite ten items and I want you to recall as many as possible in the right order." Alice had no problem with this, because she had always used her set of associated images. This involved learning a set of words rhyming with the numbers one to ten (bun, shoe, tree etc) and linking them with the ten new words – the more bizarre the connection the better from the point of view of recall - and, of course, you could quite easily retrieve the words in random order.

"Now you have to subtract numbers: what's one hundred minus seven? Now take away another seven. And again. Once more, seven off. And one final time gives you?"
"My pension, hopefully," said Alice.
"And just to check your memory again, what were the ten items?"
"Easy," said Alice, and reeled off the list, like an actor after the umpteenth performance of a speech.
"Next, it's your language skills," said Matthew. "What is this item called?" holding up a sieve.
"It's a round thing with holes in it," said Alice, "a bit like my memory."
"And now, repeat the following after me: "If a constraint be applied to a system in equilibrium, the system readjusts to nullify the constraint." Matthew thought for a while.

---

[30] MMSE: The Mini Mental State Examination (abridged)

"Could apply to my recovery, ***Le Chatelier's Principle***," he said. Then he proceeded to get Alice to follow instructions both spoken and in writing, then get her to write a sentence and finally to reproduce a complex geometrical figure.

"So how well have I done?" asked Alice.
"Twenty-four out of thirty," replied Matthew.
"That's a relief," said Alice, "So I'm ***compos mentis***, then, I assume?"
"It says here you fall into the category of mild to moderate impairment. Probably worth buying one of those 'mind games for morons' books," said Matthew, "But you see how it's a case of ***There but for Fortune***, don't you?"
"Indeed, I do," said Alice.

"So what do you intend to do about this lamentable state of affairs where individuals' fates are determined by the toss of a dice?" asked Alice.
"Well, I know I can't achieve anything alone, no matter how loud I shout. I think there's safety in numbers and, as they used to say in solidarity, unity is strength," said Matthew.
"Single issue politics can be quite effective nowadays," said Alice, "especially if you make judicious use of the internet to promote your cause; but make sure, when you have a quiet word with the professionals, that you talk to someone higher up the tree, if you want results. Oh, and get to know the movers and shakers: journalists, local councillors, MP's, etc."
---
Some twelve months after his episode, Matthew plucked up sufficient courage to volunteer to talk to some teenage school pupils about his experiences. Along with three colleagues placed strategically at various points along the continuum, representing everything from borderline personality disorder to schizophrenia, he gave his presentation to the assembled group. The impact was quite awe-inspiring – so much so that they had to give the kids time out to come to terms with what they had heard. However, the event was a great success, judging by the number of kids that approached them later in confidence to discuss similar conditions they were having to deal with in their own families. It emerged that some were young carers, secretly looking after psychotic parents; others were themselves going through ***episodes***, unsure whether these constituted just 'normal' teenage experiences, or fully-blown hebephrenia. It had been emotionally draining for the four performers, Matthew included. One woman had opted out at the last minute, and who could blame her? Yet, with the passage of time, and provided he was not too close to home when he did the talks, Matthew grew to be able to cope with his story in a more detached kind of way, as if the person he was discussing was someone else, not himself. Occasionally, he would forget where he was and find himself getting upset on the poor child's behalf, for that is how he now regarded his former self, as an infant.

One day, the same team of speakers was asked to talk for the benefit of trainees in the field of mental health. Matthew had once again volunteered. His three colleagues stressed their dependence on medication to survive (thus showing ***insight***, in psychiatric speak) whilst Matthew was honest enough to admit that he abandoned his medication as soon as he got out of hospital.
"You've clearly been wrongly diagnosed!" barked one of the professionals, not wanting the trainees to get the wrong idea, "You can't possibly be bipolar!" Matthew was just about to thank her, sarcastically, for liberating him from a wrong diagnosis, but he thought better of it. It hurt not to have his 'label' acknowledged. Whatever else Matthew might be, he was not a fraud, and wondered if the psychiatrist would have been so quick to doubt his credibility, if ***she*** had spent a month on medication in a madhouse.

Having been on the receiving end of so much quackery, you might have imagined that Matthew would have steered well clear of attempting to diagnose and treat those with psychological illnesses; but as with so many aspects of his paradoxical existence, Matthew decided to dispense medical wisdom rather than to receive it. "It is more blessed to give than to receive," he thought to himself.

## Chapter fifty-nine – the doctor

**"I told you I was ill!"**
**Spike Milligan's epitaph**

"If you want my advice," said Anita, "you'll steer well clear of doctors and hospitals, with all the class A pharmacological drugs that they push to treat physical ailments! There's a lot of iatrogenic illness out there." Anita ran a very successful business in alternative medicines, which derived much of its success from word-of-mouth testimonials from satisfied clients.

Matthew had his own crusade. Having himself been on the receiving end of medication originally used for tranquillising horses, Matthew had decided not just to debunk the efficacy of a plethora of psychiatric medication, but to seek out for himself tried-and-tested alternatives, as well as perhaps to discover a whole new way of overcoming mental illness.

First of all, he conducted a comprehensive review of the literature, looking out for individuals who were prepared to blow the whistle on the greatest example of exploitation of the vulnerable on the planet. He read with alarm anecdotes from penitent psychiatrists who were prepared to put their jobs on the line highlighting the toxicity of some medications, and who as a consequence of having exposed the truth had lost their jobs. He was not surprised to find the majority of representatives of this profession closing ranks, but surely, if they understood their subject to any appreciable degree, they were complicit in endorsing the wholesale propagation and proliferation of substances they knew were harmful to human health, as they gratefully enjoyed the corporate hospitality and foreign holidays lavished upon them by the drugs companies? It seemed ridiculous for the latter to call for the outlawing of so-called "alternative" medicines on the grounds that they had not undergone the necessary clinical tests, when the ***happy pills*** got passed after being tested on such a small sample. The side-effects - such as violent attacks either in the form of self-harm or even, in some cases, murder - only emerged when virtually half the population of America were already taking them on a regular basis.

Matthew was quite relieved one day when he discovered that the UK government were proposing to cut back on the random prescription of psychiatric drugs. As an alternative, they were proposing cognitive behavioural therapy (CBT) and he had some time for the likes of talking therapies, but wondered how quickly the government would be able to train up the necessary counsellors. He also wondered how the drugs companies would react to this inevitable loss of earnings. Obviously, the government heralded this change in policy by putting a positive gloss on the decision, stressing their intention to espouse CBT from now on, but Matthew knew it was more about saving money and getting those on ***disabled living***

***allowance*** back to work. After all, that would save money in many ways: a reduced benefits budget, a reduced need for support workers and community psychiatric nurses, a massive reduction in the bill for overprescribed, or in some cases, unnecessarily prescribed medicines, and a chance to tax a whole new set of notionally able-bodied workers.

Matthew decided it was time to put his assumed skills as a quack to the test. Marjorie was his first medical case in 2008. The problem was she was getting diametrically opposed advice from the psychiatrists and psychologists she consulted to the messages that Matthew was giving her. They would emphasise the importance of taking the increasingly higher doses of medication, whilst he kept on telling her that many of her 'symptoms' were emanating from these very same medications.
"When you finally decide," said Matthew, "that you want to recover, you'll ditch all these artificial psychological crutches, and recuperate on your own, but until then, I suppose you'll just have to go on ***showing insight*** , and taking the drugs as prescribed."

"I'm frightened to go out, nowadays," said Marjorie, who had previously been an extrovert who liked the outdoors. Marjorie was an accomplished singer with a powerful voice and a commanding stage presence. This just did not make any sense. Matthew believed that the solution often lies in the opposite of what a person is saying, and pondered Marjorie's current situation. Here was a woman whose brain was clearly very high functioning, judging by the frenetically energetic way her mind used to function. She had a razor-sharp wit and was always on the ball when it came to repartee. Yet now she was saying that she dared not venture outside, even to the post-office.

"I think you actually need ***more*** stimulation," suggested Matthew, "certainly, not less." Marjorie was scared,
"But I can't even function properly in familiar situations with close friends," she said. "Surely, if I can't cope with that, novel experiences would totally freak me out?" Matthew shook his head,
"I disagree," he said, "I believe that very novelty would help to cure you of your current anxiety. Look how much better you were, functioning in a big cosmopolitan city as compared to your mere existence in your current humdrum village life. You need excitement! Try meeting new people and take on some intellectual challenges." Marjorie took the last of her Prozac tablets,
"Wouldn't it be great if we could eliminate depression altogether?" she asked. "Certainly not!" was Matthew's emphatic reply, remembering a similar wish had come from Anita.

Matthew left a few books and articles by eminent ex-psychiatrists and repentant registrars for Marjorie to read, so that she could judge for herself the relative efficacy of her pharmacological treatment. He also handed her a few new age toys such as the tatwa cards with which to while away the hours. Thereafter, consultations took place over the phone, with occasional potentially therapeutic ideas conveyed by text message or e-mail.

---

"So, what is your panacea for returning the mentally ill back to full health?" asked Anita.

***"Creative, re-creative, procreative,"*** replied Matthew. To explain, it was Matthew's view that to reach a stage of tolerable equilibrium (he is reluctant to identify this state with happiness, because he believes that level of nirvana cannot possibly co-exist with the real world), people should engage in creative pursuits such as art, music, drama, dance and creative writing. In much the same way, physical activity - such as sport, playing games or simply, cycling or just walking – can be therapeutic. Last, but certainly not least, comes a satisfactory sexual relationship, of course, the procreative dimension, in other words.

"And why do you believe your motto can work?" asked Anita.

"In all three of the above, the individual is preoccupied with the moment, the present. How often do we find depressed people stuck in the past or fearful about the future, never actually enjoying the moment? ***Carpe diem*** is my philosophy, as you know. When I worked with those either living with or, hopefully, recovering from mental illness, I found that in simply producing ornaments using basic papier maché , people could talk quite candidly about their experiences: something they could not do in social situations.

"But surely the ***past*** and the ***future*** need to be incorporated into their lives as well?" observed Anita, "How would you go about that task?"

Matthew thought long and hard.

"The past needs dealing with, it's true. I've seen so many folk reliving their past like a worn-out gramophone record. The psychologists seem to offer two opposing views. Either you effectively erase the past, pretending it never happened, and replace it with a better autobiography that might have been, or you attempt to bring to the surface long since suppressed memories in the hope that this will exorcise the demons."

"And the future?" asked Anita.

"Now that's always a problem for born victims," replied Matthew, "Those of us who do plan for the future have more control over our lives than they do." As we know, Matthew was not fatalistic; he believed he could interact with his environment and change the direction it was heading in. Of course, he realised that you cannot exactly predict future events unless you are a clairvoyant or an absolute despot who always gets his own way, but he could see that those with plans, and, ideally, a wad of cash, clearly had a greater stake in their future than those who were content to let others make decisions on their behalf. He learned from the architects and town planners he had met that forward thinking is the only way to achieve anything in life. Unless you have vision and can envision your idea on a grand scale, it will never come to fruition.

"The psychiatric patients need to regain control over their lives. Look how willingly they have surrendered all decision-making to the authorities. We've created a huge dependency culture. The victims depend on their medication; they depend on the State; they depend on everyone they meet for support. We need to wean them off this dependence. But I am not talking about ***independence***: many of their psychological problems are directly attributable to the isolation engendered by the dogma that stated: 'there is no such thing as society'. We all need to rediscover that we are ***interdependent*** – just as capable of giving as we are of taking. A sense of community will only come about once we stop thinking in terms of winners and losers. Once a sufferer finally realises that only he himself or she herself can be in control of his/her recovery, only then can he/she take the first step forwards. Abandoning self-obsession is generally that first step. Helping others who shared a similar predicament to myself was not only of some small solace to them – it was immensely therapeutic for me, too."
Anita agreed that volunteering had probably been a win/win experience for Matthew and his clients.
"So what is the next step?" she enquired.

Matthew chose his words carefully, not wishing to distort the message.
"It's like I said before, when we discussed the skills of a good counsellor," he began. "There has to be a significant number of options: it's no good identifying a one-size-fits-all solution. However much we may scorn alternative routes to salvation as crackpot ideas or religious self-delusion, we have to acknowledge that for some people, that is their chosen path. Even with my vehement rejection of drugs, I have to admit that for some, medication represents the only way of having a half-way normal existence. The key thing is: it must be the would-be recoverer who takes control over this decision to get better. No one will recover whilst still under the Svengali spell of the therapist. Once they plan out a series of future options complete with plans B, C and D in case things go wrong, they will be well on the road to recovery. It's a bit like planting seeds: you know they won't all thrive, but you plant them in the hope that some will come to fruition, and you nourish those that show promise."

"Speaking of nourishment," said Anita, "You were telling me all about your radical change of diet."
"Oh, yes, "replied Matthew, "I almost forgot that dimension to recovery. Did I mention that Jean-Paul had a hand in recommending what to eat and what not to eat?"
"That's a strange aspect for a ***spirit*** guide to entertain," observed Anita.

"The one thing I remember him saying, over and over again, was: 'Don't eat cereals!' Now what possible harm could cereals do? I had eaten them all my life, not knowing that Doctor Kellogg originally advocated the consumption of his famous cereals to suppress the sex urge. Apparently, they were ***de rigueur*** on the menu for his psychiatric patients. Jean-Paul was explaining how folks like me that have a propensity to go manic can have this mania exacerbated by the consumption of certain foods."
" Did you find that out whilst you were in hospital?" asked Anita.
"Yes, I did. I gave up eating my customary daily breakfast cereal and noticed an immediate change for the better. I had been getting my initial 'high' from the food, only to experience the inevitable 'low' shortly afterwards. It was also noticeable on the psychiatric wards what a high volume of strong coffee the patients consumed, and that nearly all of them were cigarette smokers. I think these are three key elements aggravating the condition – caffeine, sugar and cigarettes."

Matthew modified his diet even further, selecting essential mineral supplements as well as excluding high GI[31] foods. His medicine cabinet now included Omega 3 capsules, zinc, manganese, chromium and several other ingredients. He did not care whether they were genuinely doing the trick; even if it was just a ***placebo*** effect, they seemed to be working. There are people[32] out there who maintain that prescribed drugs only work if the patient convinces himself / herself that they are going to work. It helps, too, if the doctor's endorsement of them is convincing. Conventional practitioners should take note: telling the patient that we're going to try out a new drug, but then adding the cautionary words: 'we don't know whether it will work' might only add to its nocebo[33] effect. But it was not just Matthew's own well-being that mattered: Now he needed to heal others.

Matthew knew that people suffering from the likes of anorexia and bulimia use food intake as the one thing they remain in control over. Whenever Matthew was seriously upset about anything, the first casualty was his appetite. Anita always knew when he was stressed out, because he would just stop eating, often for days on end. He had only ever reached the ideal weight for his build in Germany, after gorging himself on the daily coffee and cakes that they consume around four o'clock in the afternoon. At all other times, he looked positively emaciated. It was precisely when he was living alone that this unintentional starvation combined with self-imposed deprivation of sleep would lead to his first episode of ***hypomania***. Perhaps it was because he was the kind of person you might describe as a control-

[31] Glycaemic Index
[32] E.g. Dr David Hamilton ( www.drdavidhamilton.com ) –please see bibliography
[33] opposite effect to placebo (harmful; ineffective)

freak that he found himself incapable of functioning in the world unless he had total control of his own environment and, almost inevitably, the environment of all those with whom he interacted.

Once he had broken free of incarceration, Matthew resolved to do all he could to dissuade people from going along with enforced medication. He was convinced there was a more suitable alternative that did not have such awful side effects.
"The problem is," said his G.P.," Your employer needs the comfort of that small sheet of paper that we call a prescription. Although, given time, you would probably recover just as well, if not more quickly, without any medication whatsoever, your boss won't accept a note from me saying: 'give him a month off work to recover and he'll be back rejuvenated'. The body is very good at healing itself – a break-down is actually a good sign. It's a sign that you have realised you cannot go on with such a stressful life, and it has just shut down in protest. Remember, 'what doesn't kill you makes you stronger.' Oh, and by the way, there are two kinds of stress – the one to avoid is ***dis***-stress; the other is healthy stress. We all need the adrenaline shot that it delivers. It's a bit like risk-seeking. Perhaps you need to go bungee – jumping or parachuting. Your life is too safe!"

Matthew reflected on these pearls of wisdom. People are only stressed when they have no say in matters. Put them in control, and the same problem suddenly becomes an interesting challenge. Why is everyone so afraid? Governments use fear to control the electorate, as George Bush notably discovered. Bullies use fear to control their victims. Banks use fear to discourage criticism. You can substitute anyone with power over anyone without it. Matthew always returned to the Bible for etymological enlightenment. He was particularly fascinated by the expression 'God-fearing' because it appeared to actually mean 'loving God'. Do we need to fear someone to a certain extent before we can show them love, he wondered. That is certainly the basis of respect, as he had learned from his time in teaching. You certainly have to earn respect – you cannot simply expect it. Even so, it helps if the learners are somewhat in awe of their teacher. As soon as the adrenalin kicks in, you have the choice of fight or flight: neither of which are much use to a teacher!

A certain amount of fear seems to be necessary for a civilisation to function effectively, for once the pillars of society collapse (as all respect for authority disappears) certain individuals run wild in the knowledge that no one can touch them. At the other extreme, where fear paralyses the population, there is no room for courage and the casualty at the end of this process is love. Society needs people to love one another – not to turn their backs on each other in contempt. Fear generates depression, both medically and financially. Courage, on the other hand, brings hope and confidence.

The interdependence of the physical and the psychological is obvious. Usually, patients will exhibit physical manifestations to accompany their psychological symptoms, if only to justify to a sceptical world that they really are ill and deserving of sympathy. These symptoms will appear spontaneously: there is no question of them being ***deliberately*** manufactured. In any case, simply feeling low can make you susceptible to every malady in the book.

---

"Now what I am going to say to you will probably come as a shock, knowing, as you do, that I genuinely empathise with you all and have always tried to get changes brought about for your ultimate welfare," announced Matthew on one of his regular visits to the Drop-in Centre, in a paradoxically patronising tone. The members were suddenly aroused from their torpor. "Mental illness is contagious – there's no getting away from it. There. I've said it, now what is your reaction?" The members seemed downcast, let down by their former champion. "Let me explain. In business, there is often offered the following piece of advice: avoid the negative. There is some research that shows how having team members with predominantly negative thoughts stifles innovation and ambition. It's all about creating energy. It's perfectly possible to arrive at a win/win outcome provided all contributors ***give*** energy to the dialogue. Imagine it like the incubus or succubus draining out all your energy. Some people are like that: they pounce on a magnanimous individual and unload all their problems, scarcely giving the kind person chance for a word in edgeways. Like parasites, they leave the encounter, afforded temporary relief, only to save up their next download for a new host. In their wake, they leave some poor but generous soul, drained of all his/her previous energy."

"What I am telling you is how to get out of your downward spirals. First of all, you need to wean yourself off your fellow-sufferers. I know this seems harsh, because these very same people have given you mutual support and become your friends. But this world you have chosen to inhabit is like limbo, a kind of no man's land. Eventually, you need to mix with "normal people" again. Otherwise, you will merely reinforce each other's insecurities. It's too cosy here and it's a tough old world out there, but you have to be brave, if you really want to recover. The microcosm you inhabit has become the norm and you have become just as institutionalised as you would have been in a psychiatric hospital."

## Doctor Matthew's Recovery Formula

***N.B. This works for Matthew, but it may not work for you. Take from it any advice that you feel is relevant. Recovery is a personal journey, so you need to write your own prescription. For you it may be religion or your favourite medication. What is important is that you come to this decision of your own accord. Otherwise you'll feel inclined to blame Matthew if it does not work!.***

**1.** Don't try to revert to your old ways after a breakdown, however much other people might like you to return to your old self. The breakdown was nature's way of telling you that your previous existence was inappropriate in some way. Invent or discover a new existence instead.

**2.** Stop playing that 'poor me' worn-out gramophone record to your rapidly diminishing circle of friends. (And who can blame them for wanting to avoid the negative?)

**3.** Enjoy the moment and make plans for the future: this will give you back control over your life. Be an active participant – not a passive recipient.

**4.** Jettison the baggage: get rid of the crap.

**5.** Remember that ***change*** is always a positive move.

**6.** Remember the motto: creative, recreative, procreative (it's a much healthier way of looking at the world).

**7.** Remember: it's better to play the joker than to be played for a fool.

**8.** Be yourself (warts and all). Forget image, celebrity and perfection. They are all worthless aims.

**9.** In the normal world, it's perfectly acceptable to have one vision (if you have several, on the other hand, you will no doubt get sectioned!).

**10.** There's a very fine line between imagination and fantasy. Are you sure you can tell the difference?

**11.** Reduce your dependency (on drugs / people/ etc) and become more ***inter***dependent..

**12.** Try not to spend too much time in the sole company of fellow-sufferers (It seems counter-intuitive, but crazy thinking patterns can be quite infectious, as Matthew knows to his cost; a regular dose of the 'normal world', on the other hand, can be therapeutic).

**13.** Maintain a healthy diet: lots of fruit and vegetables, oily fish [a good source of omega 3]. Make sure you are getting plenty of the B vitamins.

**14.** Avoid the following (if you can summon up the will power!):

- Sugar
- high GI foods
- Tobacco
- Caffeine
- Cannabis (and most of the other drugs for that matter – whether recreational or prescribed drugs)

## Chapter sixty – the weatherman

Matthew identified closely with the users of the Centre, because, like them, he had felt excluded from society at certain times in his life, but often, it is only by being in the outside world that you can truly see what is going on in your own country.

***The barometer says changeable: give it a tap,***
***Perhaps the depression is lifting.***
***The white witches are casting sunny spells.***
***As the heat-wave arrives, will I have a brainwave?***
***Or as the hurricane approaches, perhaps a brainstorm?***
***Lightning reactions to thunderous applause,***
***High pressure sales of parasols and umbrellas***
***Satisfy my need for protection from the elements.***
***I emerge from beneath a cloud and count to eight***
***Before I ascend cloud number nine, or was it seven?***

***JS/2005***

"It can't be a coincidence," said Matthew, "that the words we use to describe the weather seem to mirror our moods." Iain, the community psychiatric nurse, sighed,
"I thought we were about to engage in some comforting but meaningless phatic communion about the weather. You know, people usually talk about the weather because it's not a contentious subject: it's just a way of acknowledging the existence of another human being without straying into exchanging personal information. But oh no, not for you, you have to turn even the weather into a psychological study!"

"But you must have noticed how the moods of your patients at the Centre change along with the weather?" Matthew persisted.
"When the loonies get over the moon," said Iain, "they might, for all I know, be on cloud nine, as you say." Matthew really wanted to engage with Iain on this topic,
"It's an acknowledged fact that SAD[34] impacts on them in the winter months; is there any evidence of high temperatures, long hours of daylight or prolonged dosed of sunshine having an effect during the summer months?" he asked. Iain smiled,
"We rarely get those conditions up here, so I wouldn't like to even hazard a guess." Matthew wanted to pursue his theory further so he tried another question,
"Is there evidence from abroad about the effects of hot summer weather?"

---

[34] Seasonal affected disorder

Iain had come across a number of studies, but urged caution before jumping to any conclusions,
"Just as you bipolars appear to be affected by SAD in the winter, there are indications that you might exhibit ***hypomania*** in the summer months," said Iain. Matthew smiled, "With me the hypomania appeared in January, how do you account for that?" Iain laughed,
"Perhaps you're always the exception that proved the rule," he said, alluding to Matthew's mischievous delight in playing the maverick.
"And suicide rates," said Matthew. "Have you looked at any studies recently?"

Iain had been involved in the analysis of UK figures and was alarmed to see the increased number of young males in the statistics,
"Perhaps it's because they've no role models today. No male figure in their own community they can look up to, emulate or learn from. Just footballers and other stratospheric celebrities," said Iain.
"And do these suicides occur more frequently at times when the weather is bad?" asked Matthew.
"Actually, no," said Iain. "This may surprise you, but the suicide rate often increases when it's hot and sunny, and these are not generally regarded as ***bad*** weather patterns."
"How do you account for that?" asked Matthew.
"There could, of course, be other contributory factors, like seeing other people enjoying themselves, or being under the influence of too much alcohol, but it might just be the fact that good weather is generally accompanied by high pressure," said Iain.

"In most countries in the world," said Iain, "the suicide rate amongst men is up to five times higher than amongst women. Which do you imagine is the only country with a higher suicide rate amongst women than men?"
"No idea," replied Matthew.
"It's China," said Iain.
"Is there evidence of a higher suicide rate in more northerly latitudes?" asked Matthew.
"The former soviet states are high on the list, and the move away from communism may have played its part, there. Particularly with older citizens who had expected to be looked after by the State, and who suddenly found that the principles they'd been taught to value were suddenly irrelevant when the formerly taboo Western capitalism became king, even in Russia.

"Do you believe in astrology, Matthew?" asked Iain.
"Well, Iain, the police tell me they arrest quite a few of our kind when there's a full moon," said Matthew. "It's supposed to be the effect of the moon pulling on the water in our bodies – and a high percentage of our body is made of water, after all – just like the moon causes the tides. It

seems a fair assumption that the sun and planets might have at least a comparable effect."
"You - like me - enjoy the sun, don't you, Iain?" said Matthew. "From my teenage years onwards, I practically worshipped the sun, enjoying its rays whenever I got the opportunity."

"You were once a teacher," said Iain, "how did weather patterns impact on the kids' behaviour?" Matthew thought back to his days on playground duty.
"It was the wind that seemed to affect them most. They went wild - practically feral, come to think of it – whenever the winds got up. There was no way of settling them down.
"How were they during a heat wave?" asked Iain.
"I think the Germans have the right idea: they send the kids home once the temperature gauge goes above thirty degrees. The British always soldier on, despite kids flaking out and suffering from dehydration. You didn't even use to be allowed to take bottles of water into the classroom in my day," said Matthew.

Matthew was keen to explore the impact of thunder and lightning, tornados and hurricanes on the mental state of Iain's patients.
"Are your patients mainly suffering from severe weather phobias, or do some of them actively seek out such weather patterns?" asked Matthew.
"There are those who developed a phobia after someone they knew got struck by lightning, of course, that's perfectly understandable, and others who acquired the phobia by experiencing a bad association with something else that was going on in their lives at the same time as the thunder occurred," said Iain. "However – and you may be one of this group, Matthew – there are others who actively seek out such weather features, maybe because they derive pleasure from the buzz or excitement generated by the imminent danger associated with such phenomena."

"My grandparents always went through an elaborate ritual if a thunder storm had been forecast," said Matthew. "They would cover all mirrors, knives and other metal objects with cloths or blankets, and, as the storm approached, they would open the front door." Iain was puzzled,
"I can see the dubious science behind taking superstitious measures to avoid the lightning being offered conductivity, but why open the door?" Matthew grinned,
"To allow the thunderbolt that Jupiter hurled down the chimney to escape, apparently!"

"Have you ever considered doing my kind of work yourself?" asked Iain.
"Well," said Matthew, "since you ask, I have toyed with volunteering, but I want it to make a real difference, and I don't think I can achieve that at the Centre." Iain had a suggestion.

"Why don't you volunteer for advocacy? I'm sure you'd be able to empathise with the individuals very well, having been through the same experiences yourself." Matthew decided to become an advocate, and was to gain an unexpected insight into how the various higher authorities operate. Suddenly he was thrown in face-to-face with the very bankers, lawyers and psychiatrists that he had been lampooning in his poetry; but far from being daunted by their assumed power, Matthew found himself, for once, speaking up when he disagreed with their opinions. He could never have done that on his own behalf, but in advocating for someone else, he found that his dissenting role now had a distinct purpose.

## Chapter sixty-one – the advocate

The judge was quite emphatic:
"You will have to represent clients whom you find revolting, disagreeable, stupid, naïve, pathetic, dangerous, stubborn and aggressive. You can forget your role as peacemaker and intercessor. Your role is not to achieve a compromise or an accommodation. Your role is to put the best possible gloss on your client's case without unduly distorting his or her sentiments. Remember, you are merely their mouthpiece. It could be that they don't have the appropriate vocabulary to get their point across: you can translate their Anglo-Saxon expletives into acceptable Latinate euphemisms. If a nervous reaction in court induces silence on their part, you can transcend their consternation by speaking for them. Just your presence by their side may be enough to give them sufficient confidence to speak; they'll realise that it's not just them alone versus an array of professionals and expert witnesses – you represent their ***army***."

Playing advocate of the devil had been a useful preparation for this kind of work. It had enabled Matthew to imagine how it might feel in the shoes of his opponents. He taught his students to do the same.
"Remember," he said, "anticipating the arguments of your opponents puts you one step ahead of them." (One group had to argue the merits and demerits of nuclear power, and in predicting the likely polemic, they had organised counterarguments to be available at their fingertips.) Matthew had, in any case, always been a bit of a ***fence-straddler***, so he could usually see that both sides had an equally good case, but he had to admit that he did enjoy the art of winning an argument, especially when it was either a cause he cared very little about, or, even more controversially, one where he actually shared the opinions of his opponent.

"Why do you do this kind of work?" asked Kate, his daughter. "How can you possibly want to stand up for people whose whole world view you are at odds with?" Matthew attempted to demonstrate his ***modus operandi*** to her.
"It's not for me to judge these people; I'm only the advocate. What I personally believe shouldn't come into the equation at all. I must admit that there are certain cases that I will not – on principle – take on."
"For example?" asked Kate.
"I'm not prepared to help folk just to milk the system for all they can get, when they're not prepared to contribute anything in return, not even out of enlightened self-interest."
"That's rather judgemental on your part, isn't it?" said Kate.
"It's just that I couldn't sufficiently divorce myself from those thoughts to be able to represent them fairly," said Matthew.
"Are there any others you wouldn't take on?" asked Kate.

"People I know personally," said Matthew, "you can so easily end up with a conflict of interests, so I steer clear of such cases."

Kate was quite sceptical about the efficacy of this kind of voluntary work. She herself had worked for the Samaritans as well as for a number of other voluntary groups, so she was coming at the subject with considerable personal experience.
"So what tangible evidence do you have that you've achieved anything by investing so much time and effort in advocacy?"
"It's hard to give facts and figures, because the very nature of our work is confidential, but we do always get some feedback from our head office. The main achievements are not the kind you can enumerate. It's the subtle change in attitudes we are seeing."
"How are the authorities any different now from how they were before you started?" asked Kate.
"Well," said Matthew, "For one thing, we don't get that hackneyed sentence 'this is the way we've always done it'. And another thing, they've started to acknowledge the physical presence of our client, at long last! Can you imagine what it must have been like before, with professionals ignoring the patient, speaking past her, bamboozling her with psychobabble, or, in a vain attempt to sound caring, asking her key-worker, 'Does she take sugar?' The fate of the victim had been decided long before the meeting. At least now, there is an opportunity to influence the outcome."

"Aren't you worried that your clients will grow to depend on you, rather than learning to stand on their own two feet?" asked Kate.
"What? You mean I end up needing them as much as they need me?" asked Matthew. "Yes, you'll have heard of co-dependency issues?" said Kate. Matthew had a secret chuckle to himself at this point.
"There's a constant flow of clients, and we deliberately rotate the cases within our team, if there are likely to be ongoing issues with one individual. It's all about weaning them off you from the very start. It's similar with adults who have literacy issues. I suppose it's human nature to want to ***build*** a relationship, as opposed to nipping it in the bud."

"A bit like a one-night-stand?" asked Kate, somewhat scathingly. Matthew thought through the analogy and decided to see if he could prevent its inevitable breakdown. "I'm sure you'll be surprised by my answer, but yes, in a way, quite similar to a one-night-stand. Here's the scenario: woman becomes depressed after her husband neglects her and they stop making love. Woman has brief secret affair with man who, like her, has no desire for any long-term commitment. Woman's self-esteem is restored. Husband suddenly finds her new persona attractive, regains his libido and they both live happily ever after."
"So what about the poor bloke who was exploited just so that she could get it on with her husband again?" asked Kate.

"As I said, he was a willing participant with no intentions of any long-term commitment," said Matthew.
"But it could all have turned out disastrously, you must see that?" said Kate. "The wife could have been facing a dilemma as to which man she loved, and what about her kids, how would they have felt about the affair? And we haven't even mentioned potential pregnancies or STI's."

"Okay," said Matthew, "Bad analogy. Perhaps you could supply me with a better one? Maybe one of your facebook friends could oblige?"
"You'd better not be implying that all my real friends are imaginary," said Kate. "I've acquired some really supportive confidantes via the internet."
"Sounds like a bit of a contradiction in terms, that," observed Matthew, thinking how public people's inner feelings were becoming these days.
"Better to have imaginary friends than imaginary enemies – by the way, how's the ***paranoia*** these days?"
"Touché!" replied Matthew.
"People come and go in cyberspace," said Kate, "so you can't ever become dependent on one person for advice, but there's the power you get from the numbers of people involved. If you have a problem, you can be sure that at least one of a myriad of friends will come up with an appropriate solution."

Matthew moved on to a particular bugbear of his.
"Some folk are much too proud to claim everything they're entitled to, and you really feel for them, when you hear how they've been threatened with the removal of the few benefits that they have managed to get. You sit with them for three hours filling in the claim form. Anyone in their situation would have abandoned the whole process after one hour, and bear in mind, an advocate is reasonably intelligent and conversant with the vagaries of the benefits system, so you're left with the conclusion that the form's probably been deliberately designed to deter claimants from making successful claims. The process of attrition gradually wears them down and most potential claimants eventually just give up," said Matthew.

"It's their health that suffers through this bureaucratic nightmare," said Kate. "They get an intimidating letter on the Friday, fret all weekend about having to turn up at the job centre on Monday, whereupon they are asked, as a matter of pure bureaucratic routine, you understand, what kind of work they are able to do. 'My client shouldn't have been asked to report here' I would say, 'she can't physically walk more than ten metres.' And they will callously remark, 'so how's she managed to get here then? She must be faking it.' I'm incensed: 'Sheer bloody will-power,' I say, 'wouldn't you be inclined to get up and out of your nice, comfortable seat, if you thought you weren't getting paid unless you did?' 'I'll arrange to conduct the next interview over the phone,' says the clerk, surprisingly, for a change, sounding reasonably sympathetic.

"Have you ever felt your own personal safety was at risk when meeting strangers with psychiatric conditions?" asked Kate.
"Nowadays, we're obliged not to put ourselves and, by implication, our colleagues at unnecessary risk. Meeting on neutral territory is a good idea," said Matthew. Kate pondered his choice of words.
"You say nowadays; what used to happen, then?" Matthew recalled one afternoon spent in the company of a ***paranoid schizophrenic*** whose behaviour patterns were very volatile, to say the least. Matthew's task was to help the individual in question write a letter of complaint about his treatment during one of his episodes.
"At first," said Matthew, "I could really empathise with the humiliation the guy had experienced in having his clothes pulled off him so that he could be sedated." Kate was familiar with the procedure,
"Yes, you usually have to give them an injection in such circumstances."

Matthew returned to his story.
"The situation is usually exacerbated by the fact that no one seems to be prepared to listen. And he was determined to have the letter written his way, despite my subtle suggestion that the authorities would tend to ignore any communication peppered with four-letter words, personal remarks verging on the libellous and no attention to layout, level of formality or length (this epistle/diatribe ran to nine pages)." Kate smiled knowingly,
"And how did he react to your pedantic comments?" Matthew took on board the fact that his pedantry was something that Kate herself was often on the receiving end of. "He just insisted in doing it his way," said Matthew, "And given his history of violent outbursts, I felt discretion was the better part of valour. Although I had a lap-top with me, he wasn't having any of that form of communication: he insisted that I hand-write the whole thing. 'Only official letters from nosy officials get typed,' he said, 'mine has to be hand-written.' " Kate was curious as to how Matthew survived the three hour ordeal,
"How did you manage to keep him calm?"

Matthew described the venue and the charged atmosphere their meeting had engendered.
"First of all, you're on hostile, unknown territory. You select a seat close to the door, planning your exit strategy from the start, should things go pear-shaped. The flat was a considerable distance from where I had parked the car, along a series of labyrinthine passageways. From my chair, all I could focus on was his mountain of medication, piled up for future use."
"How many different drugs?" asked Kate.
"There must have been around ten varieties. He talked about them a bit. His lay language actually put the whole issue of medication into perspective. 'This one's for bringing me down when I'm up, and this one's to counteract the side-effects of the first one. This one's to lift me when I'm down, and this one's to counteract the side-effects of that one. This one's to help me

sleep. The other five are to treat physical illnesses brought on by the other drugs: heart, kidneys, liver, that sort of thing.' When he was allowed to talk about himself, his favourite topic, he was okay."

"How did you manage to de-escalate the situation, when it threatened to be getting out of hand?" asked Kate.
"It's hard to say," said Matthew. "I kept on telling myself to keep calm and not allow him to pick up any fear from my voice or body language. When he mentioned knives, I felt this was a test to judge my reaction, so I calmly ignored the direction the conversation could have been heading. Strangely enough, I felt that it was I who was calling the shots, manipulating my marionette with my words, like administering a measured dose of morphine to a dying patient. Whenever he showed signs of kicking off, I'd switch to tranquilising text mode and find him instantly mollified."
"There you go again," said Kate, "You can't shed that control-freak image, can you? But how did you escape, in the end?" Matthew thought back to the salacious revelations he would read as a young teenager in the ***Sunday People***, where journalists left you wondering if they were really so much whiter than white in their investigations of the sex industry:
"I made my excuses, and left," he replied.

After representing a variety of clients, Matthew reached the conclusion that their plight was exacerbated by the way they were treated – or, more accurately, allowed themselves to be treated - by the assembled authorities. They reminded Matthew of the 'kangaroo court' experience that had helped to propel him into insanity. He could identify with his clients' reluctance to protest, faced by professionals who constantly disallowed comments from their victims on the grounds that his or her utterances were 'not for this meeting'. The experience was calculated to engender a 'dependency culture' that would keep the professionals in a job for life, by ensuring that the dreaded word ***recovery*** remained a deluded fantasy. He had to constantly check whether he too might be contributing to that dependency culture, as he came to appreciate some of the professionals' own personal dilemmas. Regular contact with the various teams, where colleagues become virtual friends, sometimes makes it harder to challenge virtually everything they had to say. But he was an advocate, not a mediator, in this instance, he continually had to remind himself.

Matthew had always insisted on doing things for himself. He was not only reluctant to seek help, but positively averse to revealing such a potential weakness. However, he was to find that such autonomy was, briefly, taken right out of his hands.

## Chapter sixty-two – the passenger

It was Easter, 2000. After a spell 'inside' as he put it, Matthew no longer had the independence, convenience or flexibility of a motor vehicle and had to rediscover the delights of public transport. He did not enjoy travelling long distances by bus or train at the best of times, but on medication, the ordeal was far worse. He knew he had a twelve hour journey ahead of him, including waits to meet connections, and this alone was enough to send him crazy, but he took a deep breath and boarded the early train. It was packed. For the first four hours, there were students returning to college, sitting on rucksacks, suitcases and other improvised seating arrangements, and although he did have a seat himself, having booked a reservation, the sheer claustrophobia of the experience was unimaginable. Had he been well, he would probably have coped by dozing off for the duration, but in his agitated state, all he wanted to do was to get up and walk about. At least he was not as restricted as he would have been on a bus. The mental anguish was accompanied by what he could only describe as a queasy sensation in his arms and legs that persisted the entire duration of the journey. But it was no ordinary queasiness: it was like insects crawling inside your veins, or persistent low voltage electric shocks. The last time he had experienced anything remotely like it was in Germany when he was diagnosed with ***Sehnenentzündung***. [35]

His destination was one that proved to be very popular with psychological fugitives from the rat-race. It was a railway-station in Thurso, literally at the end of the line. Whether they all found what they were looking for, he could not say, but the fact that many eventually settled there, rather than returning to their roots, suggested it offered something therapeutic. He met ex-servicemen still plagued by their traumatic experiences in the Falklands or the Gulf who talked to him the same way as Rich, one Viet Nam veteran, had thirty years before,
"I can't stand the crowds, man. They do my head in. I need to be out in the wild. I don't even need a roof over my head because I learned how to survive in the army. It's the solitude I like – it means I'm not tempted to break some poor guy's neck just 'cos he pisses me off. And the nightmares keep right on coming from those days when we went after Charlie Kong. Taking all that dope didn't help, neither. Now I don't know dreams from hallucinations." The story was the same for many of the soldiers who had served in the Gulf aged only nineteen, just like the American guy had.

Then there were those who had gone to the metropolis in search of the bright lights, found them, then rejected them in order to try and regain their sanity.

---

[35] Inflammation of the sinews

"Agoraphobia, it's called," said Simon, "but no one believes me when I say I have it, especially not the job centre. They think that only women suffer from it. It's a stay-at-home, sedentary, female kind of phobia, not one for men at all. Men are allowed to have macho fears like homophobia, xenophobia or ***gametophobia,*** of course, the fear of marriage. I'm quite happy to stay at home with my dog, and that way nobody bothers me and I don't bother them."

"Look at the sky up here, Eric," said Matthew to the film-maker. "I bet you feel horizontally challenged, after spending so much time filming in the cities with their skyscrapers. I always found those strong vertical lines obscured my vision. Just look at the panoramas up here."
"And the light," said Eric, "is just perfect for filming."
"What a lot of us like," said Matthew, choosing to be the spokesman for all psychiatric refugees, "is the magical quality of life up here. You can forget what's happening in the wider economy: that scarcely makes an impact up here. So long as you're not expecting to make pots of money, you can have a very comfortable existence. There's very little crime, lots of beautiful landscapes without hordes of tourists to spoil them, minimal pollution of both the noise and environmental kind, fascinating flora and fauna; and we get our fair share of culture from touring companies, whether it's opera, ballet, theatre, or any other art form."

Johnny protested,
"That's all very well for you well-heeled middle-class types, but the rest of us don't get a look in." Matthew wanted cultural and leisure activities to be available for all, so had been instrumental in putting on charity music events for his friends, free of charge.
"I've seen you at some of the gigs, Johnny, and I know you've contributed to poetry readings yourself."
"Yes," said Johnny, "but it's the transport costs that are so prohibitively expensive, and the buses are either very infrequent or non-existent. Did you know the taxi fare from ***out west*** is over twenty pounds?"

"So it's a bit of a mixed blessing, is it?" asked Eric. Matthew thought for a while before answering,
"I prefer to stay close to the town, but if you want true isolation, you can go and live way out west, if you prefer. Of course, you have to take on board that transport is a real issue in remote rural regions."
"And what appeals most to you personally about this existence?" asked Eric.
"Living on the edge," said Matthew, without hesitation. "For one thing, I love the challenge of the extreme weather conditions. The uncertainty that snowdrifts and force ten gales bring. And there's that Celtic legend about entering into another world where the land meets the sea. Then there's the practically universal tolerance of eccentricity up here. Most of the folk who

add to the colour of our community through their peculiar ways would probably be locked up if they behaved that way in the city."
"Yes," said Eric, "successful economies don't like to carry 'passengers', as they call the folk they don't believe to be contributing to the prosperity of the company: they're looking for drivers, not passengers."

## Chapter sixty-three – the driver

***"You, you're driving me crazy!"***

"We get a lot of them, up here in the Highlands," said Dr Scott. "Folk who don't plan ahead. They underestimate the distances and time involved in driving the length and breadth of the UK. Consequently, assuming they haven't fallen asleep at the wheel, they end up totally ***hyper***."
"Why's that?" asked Matthew.
"Well," said the psychiatrist, "it's the fact that they often set off in the evening with the perfectly logical excuse that they'll avoid potential traffic jams that way, but having deprived themselves of sleep, as every soldier knows, they start exhibiting signs of hypomania, and sometimes it gets so bad that they have to be sectioned in their own interests, as well as those of other motorists and society in general."
---
After a trip to the island of Skye had been mooted, Matthew volunteered to drive the minibus, but he had not fully appreciated what effect it can have on people with mental health issues when their normally banal but predictable existence gets disrupted. Just the break in routine would be enough to generate overstimulation, but combine that with the notion of a summer holiday in residential accommodation and the eight hour drive to get there, and you have mayhem. Frequent toilet stops had been carefully planned ahead, but when one young lady demanded he stop for something she urgently required from the pharmacist, Matthew went out of his way, making a major detour to reach the town, assuming medication was the issue. It transpired that what Kitty needed was 'emergency cosmetics' in the form of lip-stick (hardly an ***emergency***, in the circumstances!)

Another snag when gaining your minibus licence is that you are in demand to convey all kinds of groups around. When he took a group of assorted musicians on a jaunt, Matthew was surprised to find cars honking and flashing their lights as they passed him. Only later did he learn that the musicians in the back had been mooning at passing motorists. The bus needed a thorough clean-up after this trip, partly to clear away any evidence of illegal substances having been consumed, and he resolved not to transport groups of musicians ever again.

Driving the seven-ton Mercedes truck, on the other hand, had been quite an adventure, back in 1976. There was a powerful spring beneath the accelerator so that if you fell asleep at the wheel, the lorry would automatically grind to a halt. Richard and Matthew took it in turns to drive from Germany back to England, getting the strangest looks from Brits who thought this was a German invasion – the lorry being a pre-WW2 Mercedes model. Getting a puncture was the last straw in an already action-packed journey as far as having to produce the required documentation at sundry border-checks. However, a garage obliged with a lorry-jack, and, after a short delay, Matthew and Richard managed to change the wheel.

---

The point about driving is that it puts you in control, and people with ***drive*** are well motivated. Being a passenger takes all that control away from you, and you are dependent on others for the success or otherwise of your venture. Matthew taught Kate and Mark to drive when they were thirteen, trusting that it was better to make sure they could handle a car, if ever the need arose. Both of them got practice – provided by a driving school, in conjunction with the school - on the skid-pan where local bus drivers usually did their training.

When you drive, it puts you in control – a situation with which Matthew always felt most comfortable. That same instinct of wanting to be in control manifested itself in Matthew as the vice, as some people would see it, of needing to manipulate both people and situations to suit his own will. Matthew, having honed the skill over a lifetime as an alternative to achieving fighting prowess, regarded it as a virtue.

## Chapter sixty-four – the manipulator

"NLP - It's a dangerous weapon in the wrong hands," said Hazel, when she realised Matthew was trying it out on her.
"I totally agree," said Matthew, "Don't you think it would be advisable for both of us to lay down our arms? We Virgos need to stick together."
"I don't see us having remotely anything in common," replied Hazel, "Look at your desk, you're so disorganised. I thought Virgos were supposed to be perfectionists!"
"That's what makes us so critical of others," retorted Matthew, "We have the ability to analyse a problem and immediately see how it can be fixed, but it's that moat and beam hypocrisy again, isn't it?"
"How do mean?" asked Hazel.
"We're so busy seeing the faults in others that we fail to see the very same faults in ourselves." said Matthew.

Hazel needed to rethink her strategy, knowing that Matthew was alert to techniques such as mirroring to get the person on side. Why was Matthew always so obtuse? Did he deliberately set out to alienate people? Why didn't he just go with the flow and ingratiate himself like everybody else? She was curious to know the answers to these questions, but unsure how to ask them in such a way as to get a straight response. "Matthew," she said, engagingly, "do you mind if I ask a question?"
"It depends if it's a straight question," said Matthew, "but go ahead." Hazel paused before posing her question. Then after an explanatory preamble, she came out with it: "You always get shot down whenever you put forward your controversial points: hasn't that taught you to keep your big mouth shut, just in the interests of self-preservation? Are you just basically a masochist?"

"That's two questions," said Matthew, "but at least you came straight to the point. Now, here's an honest answer. You may find the technique useful at some later date. The reason I raise these issues is to stimulate debate."
"But all possibility of debate is immediately stifled once your point has been dismissed out of hand," said Hazel.
"Not entirely," said Matthew. "You see, I've sown the seed of doubt. The powers-that-be will go away and mull it over, perhaps coming to see the situation with a fresh pair of eyes. Next thing you know, my germ of an idea will be heralded as company policy, endorsed by management."
"But you don't get any credit for coming up with the idea!" said Hazel, wondering what possible motivation could be driving Matthew.
"I'm not precious about ideas; I can always come up with plenty more. In any case, I wouldn't really be interested in following them through. It's for others to dot the i's and cross the t's.

"It's the same with information. I don't like to sit on it in a vain attempt to boost my illusion of power; I prefer to share information."
"Yes," said Hazel, "we've noticed." Matthew immediately picked up on the less than subtle change of pronoun from ***I*** to ***we*** to create an 'us and them' scenario where Matthew was by implication being accused of not being a good team-player.
"Look, Hazel," said Matthew, "we both know that all of us have a tendency to be indiscreet occasionally, but I'm not talking about revealing confidential, commercially-sensitive information to our competitors, either deliberately or accidentally. I'm talking about the value of debate before decisions are made. Sharing information has at least two positive outcomes: for one thing, the individual has been consulted and is therefore more likely to go along with proposed changes than they are when change is imposed upon them. Secondly, management avoid facing disastrous consequences just because they have refused to run their ideas past other people, believing themselves to be infallible in finding solutions to problems."

"Why don't you exploit all your psychological knowledge? You know how to manipulate people. You could have them eating out of your hand," said Hazel. "Basically, because it would be too easy," said Matthew. "I prefer to risk alienating people and, if you like, take an artistic route."
"Whatever are you on about now?" asked Hazel.
"Drama. What's the basic ingredient of drama?" asked Matthew.
"Let me see, now," said Hazel, "could it just possibly be ***conflict***?"
"Precisely," said Matthew. "Conflict is at the heart of all human interaction, and unless you're prepared to do battle, you might as well skulk off with the other cannon fodder into the ayes or nays divisions, just because the whips told you to do so."
"That's the problem with our management, I suppose," said Hazel, "They're all ***shapers*** with the obligatory whips."

"And yet, I don't see the point of incessant conflict," said Hazel. "Surely, it would be better for everyone (and engender harmonious coexistence) if only people kept to the system?"
"All systems atrophy once they pass their sell-by date, which, in this rapidly changing world is before the ink has dried on the new policies," said Matthew.
"But our systems are dynamic," protested Hazel, "They're live documents, updated on a weekly basis."
"But it always ends up being like a cosy club with a privileged elite, doesn't it?" asked Matthew. "For any substantial change to occur, it needs someone from outside of the clique to come in and radically change procedures."
"I don't know," said Hazel, "Haven't we gone through enough disruption recently? I think we could do with a rest from all this change."

"You feel that way, in part," said Matthew, "because the change has been imposed upon you. Change can be truly liberating and exciting, if you embrace it wholeheartedly. Change is always better than paralysis."

"It sounds to me like you're adopting the persona of the devil," said Hazel.
"Who me? Saint Matthew, the devil? What a diabolical allegation!" said Matthew. "You always seem to want revolution," said Hazel, "Wasn't that said to be one of the devil's roles?"
"If the cap fits, I'll wear it," said Matthew, "but you must understand, I'm not about to destroy all the edifices and institutions in this world without having first ensured there are better alternatives in place."
"I've noticed how you operate, Matthew," said Hazel. "You quietly beaver away at a project, not letting anyone else in on it until it's too late to change things, and then you present it as a ***fait accompli***: what happened to your claim to want to share information?"
"It's the only way to get things up and running," said Matthew, "democracy can be so dilatory, don't you find? If I waited for permission to proceed at every juncture, my ideas would never see the light of day or come to fruition. Consultation is only acceptable in small doses."

"How do you perceive senior management, Matthew?" asked Hazel,
"Like Kevin," came the response.
"You'll have to elaborate," said Hazel, "I don't follow."
"You know, the character Harry Enfield used to play. Management are like recalcitrant teenagers and as such need similar treatment. Take reverse psychology, for example."
"Yes, I've tried that on my kids and it does seem to work. If you really don't want them to do something, you pretend you're very much in favour of it?"
"That's right," said Matthew, "And conversely, if you do want them to take a particular course of action, you argue for the opposite of what you actually want, in the certain knowledge that, because ***you*** were the messenger, the management are certain to reject the message, because they'd never want to acknowledge that any idea of yours was worth supporting," said Matthew.

"And it's the same with discipline. You go out of your way to praise any good ideas they come up with, Skinner's ***positive reinforcement***. Or more calculatingly, you adopt Skinner's ***intermittent reinforcement*** to ensure they don't get complacent about receiving your support every time."
"And how do you punish them?" asked Hazel.
"I leave it to management to mete out the ***negative reinforcement***, which, as we all know from Guantanamo, is counterproductive. My policy is to tactfully ignore bad behaviour, since I don't have any sanctions - privileges or suchlike - that I could withdraw."

"You should have been a politician," said Hazel, not wholly in jest. "You'd be very convincing in media interviews."
"Funny you should say that," said Matthew. "I don't know if you're aware of this but I've just been to Edinburgh for some media training. It's really good fun to learn how ***not*** to answer questions. We were put through the mill with the interviewer going out of his way to put his own negative slant on our story, before we'd even opened our mouths. The trick was to take the interviewer's words from his question and transform the question into what you would have liked it to have been. We were encouraged to study our script which consisted of ten key messages that we needed to get across, come what may. If we managed to sneak in five of these, we were doing pretty well."
"So how did you turn a negative into a positive?" asked Hazel.

"The initial question," said Matthew, "implied that my colleagues hadn't been very supportive. At first, I thought, how's he got that idea? I've never made that comment in any of the advance publicity information. Then I got it. I had a choice. Either I could be lead by the nose down a blind alley which encouraged me to wallow in self-pity – the emotional triggers were already set in motion – or I could use the question as a prompt for the first key message I had on my list, the importance of friends and colleagues in giving emotional support. Let's just replay the interview." Matthew popped a DVD into the player and pressed play.

"So Matthew," began the interviewer, "It seems horrendous to imagine how callous your colleagues were after all you'd been through, how did that impact on your mental health?" Matthew side-stepped the question, ignoring the pain that it could have engendered, and responded as follows:
"I think it is crucial to have the support of good friends and colleagues at times like these, and mine couldn't have been more supportive. When you're down, you don't want folk to come up with miracle cures, you just want them to be there. And by just being there for me, they have ensured that I am one of many who can and ***do*** recover from mental health problems." Matthew paused the DVD.
"Did you notice how I turned the question around?" he asked. Hazel nodded, realising that 'manipulation' was actually one of Matthew's talents, in this case, and the word need not always be ascribed with negative connotations.

Paolo, the media-man, had commented on the rich tones of Matthew's voice, deeming it eminently suitable for radio. Though he could cope with being videoed, Matthew instinctively knew that he did not come over quite as well via this medium, lacking the necessary telegenic sparkle. Matthew did, however, think he might have made a reasonable stab at journalism.

## Chapter sixty-five – the journalist

Matthew was a ***dilettante*** when it came to working in the media. He had had letters published in the ***Times Educational Supplement*** and written reviews for Arts publications. He had done interviews for local radio stations and written articles for the local press, but that was about the sum total of his involvement. He could see how the press were at once reviled and admired – reviled for the invasiveness of their investigations, leaving family relationships devastated in their wake, and admired for their courage in standing up against villains, fraudsters and corrupt politicians.

One day, as he was casually leafing through his copy of the ***Daily Mail***, an article about Alzheimer's caught his eye. It was particularly engaging for him since he recognised the family in question, as he lived close by. As a writer himself, he appreciated the author's desire to expose the true facts of living with elderly relatives who had the disease, but on the other hand, he asked himself whether he could have brought himself to identify a relative by name and go into so much personal detail about her.

"You know how much more effective a book can be when it's about real people, don't you, Matthew?" said Andrea. "Remember when they asked you whether you wanted your testimony to be anonymous or not, how you agonised over that decision?"
"Yes," said Matthew, "I never had a problem about identifying myself as a person with mental health issues: it was more about how my family might be subjected to bullying or ridicule, but now they are all grown up, I don't see it as a problem any longer."
"But isn't ***your*** novel autobiographical? First novels usually are." Matthew had thought long and hard about disguising his characters, but realised his readers were quite capable of putting two and two together. Nevertheless, he resolved to deny any intention to make his characters identifiable: if people wanted to imagine they were in his book, that was up to them. He actually felt that many of his characters had universal qualities, as well as idiosyncrasies, to which anyone might relate.

"I hear you put your own mother in a home?" said Andrea, trying to get Matthew to anticipate the ***pot and kettle*** scenario.
"I was fortunate to have had a mother who was very much ***compos mentis*** till her dying day," said Matthew.
"So why did you put her in a home? Couldn't you have cared for her in your home?" asked Andrea.
"Not really," said Matthew. "My weekly visits to her sheltered accommodation were taking their toll on my family, in any case, and I think bringing her into our home would have been the wrong decision for all concerned." Matthew held up his copy of Andrea's book.

"How did your family react, when they read the article in the paper?" Andrea was quite open about the way they were offended by such intimate details appearing in print, but justified her choice to go ahead regardless,
"If my book ensures that one family is better informed about the likely prognosis after diagnosis of Alzheimer's in a relative, I'll feel it's been worth it. That way, they'll avoid making the wrong decision."

"So tell me," said Andrea, "what's your crusade all about?"
"I've been careful to avoid that word," said Matthew, "I prefer to call it a campaign." "But, however you decide to name it, you're trying to change attitudes, am I right?" "You can try to inform people till you're black in the face, but will they listen, no," said Matthew.
"There's none so deaf as those that will not hear," said Andrea, modifying Proverbs ever so slightly.
"I tell them not to take the drugs – prescription or recreational – but they hang onto them like a crutch," said Matthew. "I tell them to stop self-obsessing and learn how to communicate with the outside world again, but they can only talk about themselves, after years of being encouraged to do just that. Could you ever imagine a single instance where they have - even for just one second - taken an interest in the personal problems of their psychiatrist? Why would anyone voluntarily reveal intimately personal information to a male or female psychiatrist who is not prepared to disclose anything about themselves?"

"Matthew," said Andrea, "you've inhabited the kind of fantasy world my mother-in-law experiences. Do you fear you'll end up like her?"
"It had crossed my mind," said Matthew. "As you approach senility, everyone jokes about your poor short-term memory, or your inability to see an object that is staring you in the face. I've always had a problem remembering names, but recently it's got much worse."
"And have your family commented about you regressing to child-like behaviour?" said Andrea.
"Personally, I believe it would be no bad thing if more people started to re-examine the world they inhabit through the eyes of a child. Only by remembering who we were as a child can we regain our true identity, after all. That multiplicity of personae we offer to the world is just like characters in a play, the dramatis personae."

"And are you ***absent-minded***, occasionally?" asked Andrea.
"Now there you have a clue as to what might be going on with various degrees of insanity," said Matthew.
"Please explain," said Andrea.
"You've heard the derogatory remark, 'she's not all there', haven't you? It is my contention that such souls are not inactive, but in fact busy acting out their lives in a parallel universe."
"Sounds a bit far-fetched, to me," said Andrea, "where's your evidence?"

"This kind of thing," said Matthew, "doesn't operate within the norms of your scientific world. You might as well ask, 'where's your scientific evidence for the existence of God?' Imagination is far more powerful than reality".
"So when my mother-in-law talks about her dead parents being very much alive, that's in a separate world that she visits from time to time?" suggested Andrea. "Could well be," said Matthew. "You often find, if you ask a medium, that she has had some near-death experience, and this has left her with unexpected psychic abilities. And if you'd ever been truly insane, you'd have coexisted in two worlds without knowing which one was real."

"So it's rather like being at a séance, communicating with the dead?" asked Andrea. "That's right," said Matthew. "But the dead are very much alive in this other world. There are some cultures in South America who set places at the table for deceased relatives. Shortly after my mother died, she spoke to us through a medium, and I was convinced she had rejoined her own mother and sisters in the after-life. Those same deceased family members were the very people we had been talking about, just before she passed away in my arms, and we talked about it being okay for her to leave us now and return to them."

"So how did you cope with drifting in and out of parallel universes?" asked Andrea. "At first," said Matthew, "it was like being an actor, with two productions running simultaneously. You'd be constantly worried about forgetting where you were in one script, but picking up a prompt from the ***souffleuse*** which set you off on a different script altogether. Another analogy might be Jekyll and Hyde, or perhaps, Walter Mitty." Just at that point Matthew noticed that Andrea had been taking copious notes. "And the title of your book?" enquired Andrea.
"You'll find that out when the novel comes out," said Matthew, suddenly guarding his ideas, realising that they were commercially sensitive. He anticipated playing the lead role in some as yet unpublished novel for which she now had the basic storyline.

"I can imagine," said Andrea, "that it would be a bit like being an interloper; not properly belonging to either world: someone of mixed race, for example, or some parvenu from humble origins suddenly elevated to the nobility." Matthew thought of another analogy:
"You know what it's like to be pushed into the swimming-pool by your so-called mates? It's a simple matter of sink or swim. Well, being 'born' into this other world is similar, only it's unlikely you'll have had any experience of how to function there. Imagine being tossed out of an aeroplane without a parachute, and you suddenly realise you have to learn how to fly, if you are to survive."

"So how do you learn to separate the two worlds – I assume there are only two?" asked Andrea.
"I can't say for sure how many are out there," said Matthew. "I've only experienced two, but some people claim there are actually eleven of them: superstring theory, and all that. It would appeal to you, there's some scientific evidence for it, you see, but I still don't believe the man working down the chip shop is Elvis, however much he swears he is. I see how you investigative journalists operate. You lure people into a false sense of security by taking an apparent interest in their favourite subject, i.e. themselves. Then you proceed to pump them for information, always on the alert for headline-grabbing exposés, or succulent quotes. A little exaggeration here and there, along with some discreet pruning of unnecessary verbiage, and Bob's your uncle, there's your story. Just the little matter of getting the editor to find a space for it."
"It doesn't work like that at all," protested Andrea.

"But isn't journalism just like writing a novel, in some respects?" asked Matthew. Andrea disagreed,
"Journalism – at least investigative journalism – is all about arriving at the truth: novels are sheer fantasy." Matthew did not agree,
"Everybody makes up stories. The degree to which my novel may be autobiographical in parts is just a matter of judgement on my part. Your version of ***the truth*** in your stories is only one person's perspective of the truth."

Andrea realised Matthew was going to have a long journey ahead of him in his attempts to write a decent novel. However, his admission that he had been put on ***haloperidol***, just like her mother-in-law, suggested he might have an insight into their shared twilight world.

## Chapter sixty-six – the writer

Matthew was sitting outside the Hotel Nacional de Cuba, drinking a Mojito cocktail, when he was joined by an 'old friend'.
"What do you have to say, Earnest?" asked Matthew.
"When writing a novel, a writer should create living people; people, not characters. A character is a caricature," said Ernest.
"The good parts of a book may be only something a writer is lucky enough to overhear, or it may be the wreck of his whole damn life and one is as good as the other," said Matthew, quoting Ernest, but it was all starting to sound like a sketch from ***Whose line is it, Hemingway?***

"So tell me," said Ernest. "Which is it? Eavesdropping as a result of indulging in the cocktail party syndrome, or the autobiography of a nervous wreck?" Matthew felt a joke coming on,
"You'd better consult the ship's doctor, if it's just the latter; but I like to think it's a combination of my keen auditory acuity as well as my life experiences."
"So who's your latest writer role model?" asked Ernest.
"Well, I have to say, I'm particularly fond of Barack Obama's work. For a politician, he's quite something. Great to have a poet in the White House, isn't it?"
"Let's see what he does about Guantanamo, first, shall we?" suggested Ernest, "It would be nice for my friends here in Cuba, if we could start trading normally with the US at some future date."

"This is the point at which you have to stop playing the puppeteer," said Roland[36], "otherwise I'll have to shoot you!"
"Come on, Roland, be fair," said Matthew, "I've aimed to present a reasonable balance between the opinions of the characters; trying to show that there are always two sides to every argument." Roland was not impressed.
"It's too self-indulgent. You're only interested in milking the reader for maximum sympathy. It's the role you've called 'the manipulator' that's coming through too prominently. Work harder on the dialectic and let some of the other characters come alive. Don't be so precious about your protagonist."

All the world's a stage, according to Shakespeare[37]. Matthew had figured in every scene of the play so far: how could he possibly adopt a low profile? Did the other characters just have walk on parts? Were they just foils or stooges, put there to show how superior Matthew was in contrast to them,

---

[36] Roland Barthes, The Death of the Author
[37] William Shakespeare, As you like it

***like bright metal on a sullen ground***?[38] It was more the case that Matthew had the ***walk on*** parts. He was the dilettante, where his interlocutors were the experts. He might have been a jack-of-all-trades, but there probably was not a single profession, trade or vocation that anyone could call him master of.

Burkhart, the German businessman, had warned him about the dangers of not focussing on one job,
"You'll never get promoted unless you devote all your attention to one profession!" Heinrich[39], offered a different perspective, although ambition probably was not at the root of that writer's advice:
"There's nothing wrong with taking a whole succession of apprenticeships – it'll give you a much broader perspective on the world and you'll acquire a far greater ability to empathise with your fellow human beings."

"What's your advice, Yorick?" asked Matthew of his friend, the poet.
"Go and read Sophocles," said Yorick, "but don't forget your roots. Stories are about people, yes, but they need to be placed in a familiar geographical setting. Where's all this action taking place? I can't detect any landmarks whatsoever. Similarly, it doesn't seem to be anchored in time. When is it supposed to be happening? Is it a contemporary piece?"

Matthew sighed. He realised that even though he was not writing a play, defying the three unities of time, place and action would be an uphill struggle, but he was determined to make it work.
"Past, present and future are intertwined in this story, so there's no sense in identifying any given point in time. The location is universal: it could be happening anywhere or everywhere, and not just in the terrestrial sense," said Matthew.

"Who are you writing for?" asked Professor Lucy Stevenson, the English specialist, "Who's your audience?"
"I suppose," said Matthew, "if I'm honest, I'm writing it for myself. Now, before you say it, I know that is the wrong answer. Before I even start to write, I have to identify my intended audience, but part of this whole process is a form of therapy, dumping all the crap." Lucy laughed,
"Not a very pleasant experience for your readers, then?" she asked.
"If I dressed it up in a more aesthetically pleasing form, I could call it 'Defragmenting the Soul'," said Matthew.
"Catchy title," said Ian, the dramaturge, leaping to Matthew's defence.

"And the audience would be…?" asked Lucy.

---

[38] William Shakespeare, Henry IV Part One
[39] Heinrich Böll

"It's aimed at professionals in the mental health industry." Lucy was puzzled.
"But you could have written an academic tome, if you wanted them to listen," she said.
"There were too many concepts that it would be difficult to back up with evidence from acknowledged authorities on the subject," said Matthew. "I feel sure I can reach a wider audience through a novel than through a thoroughly researched academic opus that gets placed on the shelves of a couple of university libraries to gather dust." "So you ***are*** targeting the laity, too?" asked Lucy.

"Isn't it a bit heavy on esoteric language for the man-in-the-street? A bit too 'Umberto Eco', don't you think?"
"That would indeed be a compliment to my writing," said Matthew. "Should I have provided a glossary, do you think?"
"No," said Lucy, "Readers like to be given the chance to look words up for themselves, if they need to. It would come across as extremely patronising, if you were to explain every polysyllabic word, as a matter of routine."
"Okay," said Matthew. "Maybe I'll just translate the Latin quotations."

"You still haven't yet told me ***why*** you are writing this book," said Lucy. "What's your ***purpose***?" Matthew had thought long and hard about this.
"It's difficult to encapsulate the purpose in one pithy phrase," said Matthew, "but I would say to persuade people to open their eyes and see what's really happening, rather than accept what they're told, regardless of the authority with which the person speaks. Oh, and love the person you are, and as a consequence you'll be able to love your neighbour, too."
"Sounds like Christ's message," said Lucy.
"Yes, I suppose it is, really," said Matthew.
---
"Can you 'take care' of my brother?" asked Harold[40]. "He's a bit damaged after the ECT, you know.
"Sounds like you're having another of your favourite conversations," said Matthew. "You know, the ones where the characters talk past one another." Harold smiled. "But don't you realise, Matthew, that most conversations are exactly like that? Communication probably wasn't the prime motivation for the dialogue of the interlocutors, in the first place." Matthew felt he was on the same wavelength as Harold.
"Is that why people engage in phatic communion most of the time, do you think?" Harold explained his own thinking on the subject.
"If you think you're on the same wavelength as me, you're most probably not," he said. "The very fact that you think you connect with me suggests you don't have much understanding of my technique."

---

[40] Harold Pinter

Not to be deterred by this somewhat disparaging reaction, Matthew tried to establish common ground with Harold.
"What gets in the way of communication, in your opinion, Harold?" he asked.
"Communication itself gets in the way of communication," replied Harold.
"You mean language; choice of words - that kind of thing?" asked Matthew.
"You don't expect me to respond with some affirming comment like 'precisely', now, do you?" said Harold. This indicated to Matthew that he was probably on the right lines. Harold added a few more ideas for Matthew's benefit,
"Silence is an excellent form of communication. As they say, it speaks volumes." Matthew could see the purity of silence, unadulterated by meaningless waffle.
"So why do so many people speak absolute crap, Harold?" Harold smiled.
"It might be because they like the sound of their own voice too much or it could be fear," he said.

Matthew considered the first point.
"I wonder if Steve, the mathematician, could help me here." Steve joined the ***online chat***, arriving almost as opportunely as Perseus. Matthew proceeded with his next joke, knowing that Steve was always a good indicator of the likely effectiveness of a home-grown joke.
"Have you tried that new laxative, Steve?" Steve humoured him.
"No, what's it called, Matthew?"
"Quantitative Easing!" Matthew replied. Harold found this example of verbal diarrhoea quite enlightening.
"See what I mean, Matthew?" he said, "why don't they call it 'printing more money', so there's no room for ambiguity, or your jokes, for that matter?"

Matthew tried to return from the ridiculous to the sublime.
"Just to make a serious point, here, Harold, if you don't mind, maybe folk need to externalise all the crap thoughts that inhabit their brains from time to time, just to stop becoming psychologically constipated. Perhaps it's unfortunate for the audience where the externalisation is verbal, but maybe if these empty vessels put their thoughts into print, the whole process could be mutually therapeutic for both author and audience?" Harold agreed:
"You could say that the readers - or audience if it's in the form of a play - have at least been offered a choice. They can vote with their feet, if they don't like what they hear, or they could pass your book onto a connoisseur of coprophilia, who might at least appreciate it."

Harold gave a gentle warning to Matthew.
"Don't imagine that if you eliminate the crap, all you'll be left with is truth. It's not like panning for gold, you know. Any nuggets you do find need to

be viewed with scepticism to eliminate iron pyrites from your panner's sample. Remember, everybody lies; everybody tells stories." Matthew knew what to look out for, "***Confabulation***, that's what the psychiatrist calls it." Harold continued,
"So it's really not surprising to find that our 'tangled web', when we come to unpick it, looks like one spun by a ***spider on seroxat***. And don't imagine the World Wide Web's any different, in that respect."

"But sometimes telling lies is quite unintentional," said Matthew. "If someone else, like a parent or teacher, for example, told you something was true, you'd tend to believe it unless and until someone came up with empirical evidence to the contrary. Take, for example, my concept of colours. If my parents happened to be marginally colour-blind, and gave me to believe that the colour we all observed was blue, I'd be reluctant to concede that it was, in fact, green." Harold had an answer,
"sixteen point seven million colours, allegedly, have been identified, so you should, in theory, be able to objectively verify whether your blue is true blue."
"I suppose the full spectrum is truly enormous, when you've taken all the hues, saturation and brilliance into consideration," said Matthew, "But thanks for the advice, I'll go and check how closely my concept of blue matches the grid."

"It's surprising," said Harold, "that any successful communication takes place at all, given the multiplicity of variables." Matthew agreed.
"There's that element of self-deception, to start with, even before the words come out." Harold developed the theme.
"Then there's the point where the speaker decides what he thinks his audience wants to hear. This probably is more about messenger than message, because he's keen to be held in some degree of esteem by his audience." Matthew anticipated the next stage. "Then there's the unpredictability of the listener. Does he hear only what he wants to hear, regardless of what is being said?" Harold added,
"Or maybe, he recalls it differently in hindsight to the way he perceived it at the time? As every good counsellor knows, you need to feed back to the speaker the interpretation you put on what you have heard them say. That way, they have the opportunity to correct any misunderstandings, and reflect carefully on how they were coming across to you."

Matthew could see how our imagination often gets the better of us, embellishing a story here and there for effect, or subconsciously misremembering a whole series of events.
"***Backwards story the tell***," suggested Harold. "You can rehearse your story, ready for a police interrogation, and sound quite plausible, but you'll find it nigh on impossible to recount the series of events in reverse order,

unless they actually happened to you. Even then, your brain can play tricks on you, misremembering the sequence of events."

"So how do you suggest I proceed?" asked Matthew.
"Remember your own most irritating characteristic?" came the response.
"Can't say that I do," replied Matthew.
"Does '***moats and beams***' jog your memory?" asked Harold. Matthew remembered how prompt he was to find fault with others; yet so reluctant to acknowledge his own failings.
"Are you telling me to refocus my critical tendencies?" asked Matthew.
"Yes, you must now redirect this carefully honed pettifogging expertise onto your own work," said Harold.

Matthew began his quest by having a heart-to-heart with his good friend, Jonathan, the critic.

## Chapter sixty-seven – the critic

**Through half-closed eyes we learn to read between the lines**
**Ideas emerging as we recognise the signs**
**Fleeting or enduring, old or new**
**Pleasantly appealing, false or true**
**The critic strives to imitate the writer's pen**
**So vainly chewing up another's words again.**

**A mystic falling-into-place, a random choice**
**Is mingled with intuitive medium's voice**
**To echo thoughts original, yet decayed**
**As out of autumn leaves a seedling's life is made**
**Without the mystery of nature's music-light**
**What ultimate provision would there be for sight?**

**And who can doubt sincerity in out own thoughts?**
**Are we just vehicles to convey cheap reports?**
**Didn't God first with an imitation begin?**
**The mirror's image surely was the start of sin**
**Reflecting on the mad ideas of crazy fools**
**Can teach us greater wisdom than we learn in schools.**

*Critically Creative Copy, JS/1969*

"You shouldn't criticise a critic," said Jonathan, "you might as well try to impress an impresario, in the immortal words of John Shuttleworth. "It's like biting the hand that feeds you. You depend on them for publicity."
"Is the relationship symbiotic or parasitic?" asked Matthew. Jonathan tried to describe the tie-in by using an analogy familiar to Matthew.
"I take it you have the services of an agent to get work for your band?"
"No," said Matthew emphatically, "we organise the gigs ourselves."
"That explains why you're always facing either feast or famine," said Jonathan.
"It's true," Matthew acknowledged, "we sometimes go for weeks without a single phone call, but at other times – and it's totally unpredictable at what time of year – we have to turn several potential venues down, because, of course, we can't be in more than one place at the same time."

"An agent," said Jonathan, "could manage that state of affairs for you." Matthew acknowledged the advantages of employing an agent, though he did not take kindly to the man taking a cut of the band's earnings,
"I don't think we could afford an agent," he said.

"If you're worried about taking a cut in earnings," said Jonathan, "think again. An agent has much better negotiating powers than you do as individuals. He has a handle on what rival bands are getting, so you'd probably find that, like an accountant, he'd pay for himself twice over."
"So how," said Matthew, "does a critic help a writer?" Jonathan reminded Matthew of his media work,
"Don't you remember that maxim, 'all publicity is good publicity; there's no such thing as bad publicity.' Notoriety is indeed - paradoxically perhaps - more ***sexy*** than fame."
"So what's the good of a crap review?" asked Matthew. "Gerald Ratner's jewels didn't sell too well after he used that avenue, did he?"
"But look, Matthew," said Jonathan, "what you're helping people to do is to clear away the crap from their lives. Don't you think that idea would appeal to most people? What you're effectively selling them is a ***turd-processor***!"

Then Jonathan returned to his defence of the critics,
"Take that line from your poem," he said. "It sounds like you're saying critics have nothing original to say?" Matthew reflected.
"You mean where I imply that critics simply regurgitate other people's opinions, I assume?"
"Yes," said Jonathan.
"But if you look at the other verses," said Matthew, "you'll see that the same criticism is levelled at the writer: nothing's ever truly original." Jonathan thought Matthew could learn a lesson from his own poem:
"As Caleb says, imitation is the sincerest form of flattery[41]," said Jonathan. "So, don't knock it. Let the critics earn their crust, too! Your very inability to handle flattery has, as its root cause, your feelings of inferiority: one minute, you're fishing for compliments, the next you're embarrassed because you don't personally think you're worth the accolades."

"Have you noticed how many synonyms there are for ***critic***?" asked Matthew.
"What do you think that tells us about the British attitude to enterprise?" Jonathan wondered. "Do you think that's why we're so risk-averse, because were conditioned to assume that 'it'll never work' or that someone is getting 'too big for their boots'?" "Yes," said Matthew, "but it's worse than that. We've all been conditioned, from a very young age, to be extremely self-critical. We're our own worst critics."
"It's true," said Jonathan. "We don't blow our own trumpets enough, like the Americans would. Instead, we're self-effacing. Boasting is a heinous crime, and we're told things like 'pride comes before a fall', so we become quite wary of sticking our necks out."

---

[41] Charles Caleb Colton

"Imagine how much better we'd all feel about ourselves if people were complimentary to one another rather than being critical, pusillanimous and damning with faint praise," said Matthew.
"Yes," said Jonathan. "Let's have more wannabes and less ***could-have-bins***." Matthew continued in this vein,
"And don't forget, criticism can be constructive, if it is offered in a genuinely helpful manner. We can all learn from our mistakes." Jonathan smiled.
"You can always tell a true friend by their willingness to take on the role of 'critical friend'. You don't want sycophants at a time when you're convinced that you're right, when everyone around you knows you're wrong. Look what happened to the banks!"
"But what good would it have done, had they told the man at the top?" said Matthew. "They'd have lost their own jobs, and Fred the Shred wouldn't have listened anyway. Look what happens to whistleblowers, even in the public sector. They get the sack for 'bringing the profession into disrepute', just for highlighting bad practice."

Having originally considered the role of critic to be parasitic on the work of the writer, Matthew started to wonder whether the relationship might, after all, be more symbiotic, with a degree of co-dependency. However much the writer might wish to indulge his flights of fancy, he effectively needed the honest savagery that the advice of his 'critical friend' unleashed on his initial efforts.
"It's in serious need of redrafting!" said Jonathan, after giving Matthew's latest chapter the most cursory of glances. "You've invented too much. It just doesn't ring true. Try basing it on actual events, rather than trying to sanitise the details to avoid upsetting folk who might only too readily identify with your characters."

Matthew decided to start afresh, focussing initially on his son, Mark, and his daughter, Kate. Another ***episode*** in his life was about to begin.

# *Episode IV*

## Chapter sixty-eight – the confabulator

Matthew imagined sitting down with his son and daughter who by now were adults with their own responsibilities.
"I was wondering if that early concentration on your education ever made you feel you'd missed out on normal childhood experiences?" asked Kate, one day, during a conversation she ***might have had*** with her brother.
"You mean like learning to read when I was two?" asked Mark.
"Yes, and I think you started operating your first calculator around that time, too," said Kate. Mark was convinced that these challenges as a child had helped him achieve very good academic results:
"We always did the reading like a game, jumping over a word as soon as I'd learned to say it. If I remember rightly, the words were printed in red, rather than black."

Mark returned to an earlier discussion they might have had.
"So, Kate, you were saying about the Christmas present..." Kate smiled, recollecting how her mother had commented on the way Mark would sit contentedly as a toddler under the stairs, with an oversized set of headphones on his head, listening to fairy tales recounted by a woman with a pronounced Texan drawl. She could still hear Mark retelling the stories, unwittingly imitating the voice, '...***but they ow-are may-a-gic bay-ans***!'
"It must have been a fantastic baby-sitting device," said Kate, "I wonder if Dad ever later regretted, having substituted the cassettes for sitting and reading to us kids, an activity which might have helped better with the whole bonding process."
"But both Mum and Dad did often spend quality time reading to us when we were kids," Mark protested.

Mark asked Kate what she could remember of ***her*** childhood experiences,
"I think I must have forgotten," said Kate. "I do remember sitting on my mother's knee, and occasionally, on my father's knee, listening to stories. I remember the pictures from the books more than the words. Mum was very ill at the time, so I may have subconsciously suppressed the memories."
Mark tried to help her recall the good times,
"You always had a really vivid imagination. I think that's why you became such a talented artist. Did you ever make up your own stories?"

Kate had to admit that she found the fine line between imagination and fantasy quite a challenge, at times.
"What's wrong with painting your own interpretation of the world to replace the one you don't like?" she said. Mark was curious,
"What was it you didn't like?" Kate reflected on the humdrum existence imposed upon her,

"I have the misfortune of being a risk-taker, a thrill-seeker, if you like. It's hardly surprising, therefore, that I found my monotonous, predictable and safe lifestyle so mind-numbingly boring; I wanted some excitement!"
"And you found that excitement in a make-believe world?" asked Mark. Kate started to get annoyed. (But then sibling rivalry is nothing new).
"There might have been the odd 'Walter Mitty' moment, but, if you recall, I always sought out hazardous activities so that I could actually experience real life rather than be constantly protected from it," said Kate. Mark recalled her driving examiner's comment: ***dangerous!*** But he decided that discretion was the better part of valour and refrained from alluding to it, in case it just exacerbated the situation .

Mark was more the cautious type of individual, at least in comparison to Kate. Like his father, he would ponder the pros and cons, as well as the potential consequences of every decision he faced, even down to the minutiae. It might be said that both he and his father exhibited 'foresight', in the words of some psychologists, but compared to Kate, the pair of them were paralysed by fear. Fear was an emotion Kate never appeared to show. Even as a child, Kate had been remarkably brave, shrugging off injections, dentistry and minor surgery without so much as a tear.

Mark wanted to explore the contrast between himself and his sister with Kate,
"You understand psychology, Kate, much better than I ever will. Can you explain the notion that schizophrenics allegedly lack 'foresight' " Kate was suspicious,
"Are you implying something here?" Mark smiled,
"Don't be so paranoid, Kate, I just wanted an explanation." Kate felt somewhat reassured,
"It is said that a recurrent symptom of schizophrenia is the inability to think through the consequences of your actions. This would suggest a complete disregard for future events."

Mark had personal experience of this:
"I tried to have a conversation with a friend (who shall remain anonymous) along these lines, pointing out to him that those who do not plan their lives ahead are doomed to being controlled by others. They become the passive victims as opposed to the active movers and shakers. Rather than shaping their own future, they are condemned to manipulation by the powers-that-be."

Kate added a further tell-tale sign of schizophrenia:
"They're prone to ***spontaneous confabulation***, in psychological terms," she said. Mark was intrigued,
"Whatever is that when it's at home?" he asked. Kate tried to put it in terms he would understand.

"If you listened to the rantings of a schizophrenic, particularly if he had just fuelled himself up on recreational medication, you'd probably glimpse fragments of logical thought. However, interspersed with these would be random embellishments, angry outbursts, wild accusations and a concoction of characters from a whole variety of worlds: you'd need to be a person familiar with ***gaming*** to recognise some of them."

Mark knew that world, but kept it separate in his head, clearly delineated away from the ***real*** reality. His affection for the work of Tolkien had taken him into a fantasy world, but he knew when to suspend disbelief, and when not to.
"Is there any way you can detect a schizophrenic from the way he tells, or retells a story?" he asked. Kate decided to recount some of her studies.
"You'll be familiar with the concept of the control group, I imagine?" Mark smiled,
"I thought that was the psychiatrists!"

Not to be deterred, Kate proceeded to describe her experiment.
"Both groups had a short story read out to them and were asked to recount it." Mark knew the technique from Germany,
"Like the ***Nacherzählung***?" he asked. Kate nodded,
"We weren't looking for a near-perfect reproduction of the original, of course; we wanted to see who recalled details from the original text and who made up ideas, perhaps to compensate for their poor skills of recollection." Mark was curious,
"So the 'liars', for want of a better word, were the schizophrenics, is that what you found?"

Kate didn't like his choice of word, but accepted that he had understood the point of the exercise.
"There were two kinds of errors, if you like: sins of omission as well as commission." Mark remembered the Lord's Prayer,
"...ought to have done...ought not to have done... And there is no health in us," he said, "remarkably prescient, those religious types, weren't they? But then, I suppose mental health teams have taken over since the Church abnegated its responsibilities in the spiritual domain."

Kate wanted to be sure Mark had understood.
"Schizophrenics made up more of their own story, rather than sticking to the original." Mark wondered if it was so unusual for people to make things up: ***romancing*** as his grandmother called it.
"Summaries are most enlightening in that respect," he said. "Unlike in your experiments, Kate, our students have the original text in front of them and are required to summarise it in their own words, using about one third of the original words." Kate was intrigued,

"If they have the original text before their eyes, that should eliminate the need for fabrication of information." Mark smiled,
"But that's the whole point, you see, Kate, it doesn't prevent our students from introducing their own ideas, and, so far as I know, none of them is schizophrenic."

Kate was puzzled,
"So you're saying that everyone is inclined to ***confabulate*** from time to time, even normal people?"
"Precisely," said Mark. "It's human nature to draw on what we already know to accommodate new information. That would account for the sins of commission, as I called them. It's especially so, where the texts are very technical, because you have to use your own words, so who can blame the poor students for putting their own embellished interpretations on the text?"

Kate ventured to add a further observation that scientists had made in the case of schizophrenics,
"We've detected a reduction in grey matter in the anterior regions of their brains." Mark could not resist the urge to get a dig at the ***sanctimonious scientists***,
"Grey matter? I thought everything was either black or white for you scientists!"

Kate and Mark were so different from one another; like chalk and cheese, really. Mark wanted a quiet life, but Kate was enthralled by a more exciting side of life.

## Chapter sixty-nine – the pyromaniac

"I'm also strangely attracted to the idea of spontaneous combustion," said Kate.
"I think I can pinpoint what sparked off that obsession," said Mark. "On bonfire nights, you were always getting your fingers burnt – through no fault of your own, you understand. Neighbours had no compunction in handing a lighted sparkler to you as a two-year-old. Not a sensible idea as we were to discover. Then we made the mistake of taking you to an 'organised' display. Someone had thrown what they took to be dud fireworks into the bonfire and, sure enough, you were on the receiving end, though luckily only your scarf (Dad's old London University scarf, in actual fact) got burnt."

"I always wanted to do the cooking on the barbecue," said Kate. "Have you ever noticed how men are quite happy to leave all the indoor cooking to the womenfolk, but once it's outdoors, it's solely their province? What's that all about?" Mark shook his head,
"I really don't know. I'm sure Dad would have let you take over. Maybe it was that protective side that males always like to show; nothing to do with their culinary skills at all." Kate smiled,
"Judging by his burnt offerings from the grill, presentation skills were clearly not his forte!"

Mark had witnessed at first hand how his farming friends encouraged new growth,
"I like the idea of burning away the old stubble and dead grass to encourage the new shoots. I feel I've done much the same thing in trying to defragment my soul." Kate smiled,
"It must be rather like getting a hair-cut." Mark frowned,
"So long as cutting the hair doesn't sap all my strength," he said, remembering what happened to Samson. "Fire for me symbolises my anger; but out of the inferno, hopefully, a phoenix can arise."

"You can't have construction without destruction," said Kate, "There's always some collateral damage. Just like having to deal with constructive criticism: not your favourite pastime, I take it,? Like being forced to take a cold shower, just when you're all fired up with ardent passion?"
"I think I get the point," said Mark.
"I like fire," said Kate, "it's full of energy. But it's not always fire that destroys, as people might instinctively assume; water, too, can be very destructive." Mark found this a perfectly natural conclusion for Kate to reach, knowing that she was a ***yin*** fire snake, whilst he was a ***yang*** water rat.
---

Matthew remembered in his student days helping to plan a demonstration, but being quite shocked by the cool, calculating way his mates talked about taking with them a supply of Molotov cocktails. Apart from anything else, he felt that these were bombs for the unimaginative: a milk bottle filled with petrol with an old piece of rag for the fuse – where is the ingenuity in making that? On the other hand, they were simple to make and generally created havoc in the mêlée. But for an accomplished pyrotechnician like himself, they were just not good enough.

Luckily for Matthew, and probably his fellow demonstrators, he was able to keep his powder dry till a later date, when the opportunity arose to create an impressive flash and resounding bang in the theatre, long before killjoys from ***hazards anonymous*** arrived on the scene. [Again, don't try this at home, kids!] It was to be an 'all singing / all dancing' production; perfectly choreographed and timed meticulously to ensure maximum effect. The band, whom Matthew had hand-chosen for their ***inability*** to read music, were perfect for the show, since they could all play by ear, and many of the tunes accompanied action in virtual darkness, with even the exit lights temporarily extinguished. There were dancers in skeleton suits, produced by applying luminous paint to their clothes; and there was strobe lighting, too. Those in the audience that hadn't already experienced epileptic fits were yet to face a surprise visit from the cardiac police.

"Careful now!" said Alan, "Just a molehill's worth of gunpowder into the bottom of the dustbin." The sorcerer's apprentice stood ready with the two bare wires at the base of the container, ready to throw the switch.
"Action!" said Matthew. With a WHOOSH! and an almighty BANG! the scene reached its spectacular climax, and to this day, the dustbin-lid remains securely lodged in the roof of the theatre, a salutary lesson to any future would-be pyromaniac, fresh from the Band of Hope! (Remember the salutary attempt at aversion therapy for seven-year-olds back in 1955?)

Matthew contemplated his rebirth. Would he arise, like Phoenix from the ashes, or would he be propelled down the birth canal, emerging into the light after spending an eternity exploring an underground labyrinth like the lab-rat he was? Childhood memories reminded him that he had been there before. Had the tunnel been a portent of things to come? Matthew needed to be underground, plumbing the depths of his subliminal mind.

## Chapter seventy – the speleologist

"Do you remember the caves, Mark?" asked Kate.
"I like the way entrepreneurs have transformed what must have been a potentially lethal occupation into entertainment for the masses," said Mark. "Just think how many mine-workers were literally dying of thirst because of the dust generated. They collected the lead-contaminated water to drink."
"On the other hand, I found the underground boat-trip pleasant, and the concert-hall was amazing." Mark had to agree,
"The subtle lighting helped. It was like being in Aladdin's Cave."
"Mind your head!" warned Anita. But it was too late. Matthew had unceremoniously destroyed a stalactite that had probably taken thousands of years to grow. A small scar remains on his head as a reminder of his inadvertent iconoclasm.

Subterranean passages remained a fascination for Matthew, despite the potential hazards that lay in wait for him. As a couple of ten-year-olds, Gary and Matthew, like the kids they grew up with, had always simultaneously feared, yet secretly relished the idea of enduring the rite of passage that was epitomised by ***the tunnel***. It wasn't exactly a railway tunnel, but it did run beneath the railway embankment, allowing a stream to pass from one side of the railway line to the other. At one time, there had probably been iron gates protecting the entrances, but these had long since been removed, so the tunnel, which snaked its way through to the other side, was a source of curiosity to the kids.
"Do you know anyone who's ever managed it?" asked Matthew. Gary claimed the local gang-leader had persuaded would-be recruits to go through, and, although most of them gave up half way through when they could no longer see daylight, one kid had emerged over the other side, terrified yet triumphant.

"Let's do it together. I'll go first," said Matthew. The tunnel was only about three foot high, so they had to walk with bent backs all the way along. There was a drought at the time, so fortunately their feet stayed dry. Once the darkness descended, they had to grope their way along, their eyes only gradually adjusting to the dark.
"Look!" said Matthew to Gary. "There's light at the end of the tunnel!" The two heroes emerged after what seemed like an eternity, bursting into spontaneous laughter, probably more as a release of the pent-up fear, than the folly of their enterprise.
---
Sue, the psychotherapist, wanted to explore the subterranean caverns of Matthew's mind.
"Have you ever noticed," she asked, "how your level of arousal varies from one day to the next?" Matthew shrugged his shoulders,

"Not especially," he replied. Sue realised she would have to set out the parameters more fully before launching into her theory.
"I take it you occasionally experience reminiscences?" she said.
"Vivid memories of events I'd thought I'd long forgotten?" asked Matthew.
"That's right, Matthew, they're often triggered by a fragrance." Matthew remembered one such example,
"As soon as I got off the train in Thurso, I was transported back to the 1950's. Do you know what caused that?"
"No idea," replied Sue.
"People burning coal," said Matthew. "After they introduced the so-called ***Clean Air Act*** where I lived, people stopped burning coal, so I've been deprived of that olfactory experience ever since."

Sue elaborated the research.
"The threshold that separates the conscious mind from the subconscious mind is never static. When you are super-awake, you can dip in and out of your subconscious psyche." Then Sue reminded him of the downside of this bipolar condition, "But there are the other occasions where you're virtually comatose," she said. Matthew explained,
"I need to recuperate after long spells of frenetic mining activity," said Matthew, about to mix his metaphors, "but the trawl is always worth the fishing expedition. I can hoover up some real gems in the process, though, I must admit, I've not had the opportunity to indulge my pastime in recent years for obvious reasons." This was an oblique reference to haloperidol, the mind-numbing medication he was taking.
"So how did you use to achieve these transcendental states?" asked Sue.
"Basically, through prolonged sleep deprivation," Matthew replied, "though a certain amount of fasting also aided the hyper-animation."

"So what was the purpose of revisiting these old associations?" asked Sue. She returned to her research into his emotions, wondering why he had always tended to suppress his feelings. "As you know, Matthew, virtually every single thing we have learnt in our lives will have had some emotional connotations. Some memories are difficult to erase because they were accompanied by painful experiences, but if it's a skill we're talking about, acquired through excruciating self-disciplinary exercise, our proficiency will remain; if, however, it's the memory of some traumatic event, it's more likely we'll have parcelled it up somewhere in the remote filing system that is our subconscious mind, so when ***you*** come across it as part of your meticulous trawl, it's like suddenly being faced with the forbidden fruit." Matthew responded,
"And I have to decide whether to leave well alone?" Matthew was convinced that ignorance was not bliss, and felt that Adam and Eve were always destined to taste the apple, "Any knowledge or discovery of knowledge can be put to evil use as well as to good use. You only have to consider the internet," he said.

"So which school of psychiatry do you subscribe to?" asked Matthew.
"What do you mean?" asked Sue.
"The one which encourages you to regurgitate all your misery, with the express aim of bringing back to life all your traumatic experiences, or the one that persuades you that none of it ever happened, and replaces the bad memories with brand spanking new memories?" asked Matthew.
"That's a rather simplistic, and if I may say so, a rather cynical interpretation of the two psychiatric techniques," said Sue, "But I see where you're coming from. To continue with my earlier image, you should carefully ***unwrap*** the parcel to remind yourself why you had felt the need to lock it away in the first place. Then you should decide whether it still represented a threat to your well-being. If it did, you should wrap it up again and replace it in its favourite location; if not, you should create a new visual link to accommodate it within your more sophisticated understanding of the world."
---
When you are young, you feel immortal. You turn away those irritating insurance people, who are desperately trying to persuade you to sign up for an endowment or pension plan. However, as you approach middle age, you start to contemplate the fact that you may not live for ever, especially when ill-health starts to get you worried.

## Chapter seventy-one – the moribund man

***morituri te salutant***

***Suetonius***

Matthew had witnessed enough deaths to realise that the immanent experience of it would not be an easy one. He pondered the predicted routes of his exit.
"What's the most likely?" he asked his friend Niall, the doctor.
"You mean now that we health professions have effectively eliminated most diseases? (always assuming you haven't made a major contribution to your own demise through substance abuse, or through neglect)," suggested Neil, trying to exclude all other potential contributory factors. Matthew believed that increased longevity was principally attributable to better hygiene, better diet and education, rather than the – admittedly - remarkable advances in healthcare.
"I maintain that environmental factors are the predominant force in the health of the nation," he said.

Niall didn't agree:
"Just tell me what conditions your parents died from, and I'll narrow down your options," he said. Matthew was not convinced.
"You're just like the witch doctors, or the gypsies with their curses," he said, "it's like a self-fulfilling prophesy: the hypochondriac within me worries so much about having a stroke or a heart attack that he brings one about." Niall acknowledged that the plagues of yesteryear had been replaced by a whole plethora of autogenously derived maladies:
"Cancer is always the favourite option, if you haven't already been dispatched by one of the other two you mentioned." Matthew wanted to make an argument against the genetics case.
"Both my parents had cancer, but why should that mean that I am any more likely to die of it. Isn't it just a matter of pure chance?" Niall smiled wryly,
"You're genetically predisposed to be susceptible to such illnesses," he replied.

Matthew was sceptical,
"But we already know that everyone has a one-in-three chance of dying of cancer, so, from purely a statistical point of view, you can't prove much of a genetic link, can you?"
"I know you're taking every precaution to avoid the disease," said Niall, "certainly eating fresh fruit and vegetables is a good idea." Matthew was keen to discover whether Niall himself took any notice of the advice to eat healthily, and, along the lines of ***Physician, heal thyself***, he asked,
"Do you maintain a healthy lifestyle, Niall?"

"None of your business!" replied Niall, to which Matthew responded in sarcastic Shakespearian mode,
"***Methinks the lady doth protest too much***." Niall promptly lit up one of his Hamlet cigars. Matthew knew that, like all professionals, medics rarely practise what they preach. Niall responded in kind,
"Clearly, the last time you died was on stage, trying to perfect a pathetic comedy routine!" Not to be outmanoeuvred, Matthew came back with a curious rejoinder,
"At least I haven't joined those 'died again atheists'!"

Humour had its place. It was therapeutic. It always has been therapeutic in helping people deal with the rather unpalatable prospect of immanent death. Matthew cogitated on the Latin verb for to die,
"It's a deponent verb, doesn't that tell you something?" he asked Niall.
"So doctors study Latin: what relevance does the grammar have?" Matthew explained.
"Death is something that is done to you (unless, that is you decide to commit suicide or opt for euthanasia). You're a victim; a passive participant without any say in the process."
"But you can choose cremation or burial," remarked Niall.
"No, that's after you're dead, I mean about the act of dying," said Matthew.
"I've often pondered this whole euthanasia business: I know when I'm faced with the choice of excruciating chronic pain, I'll probably give in and demand morphine, if some interfering kind soul hasn't already made that decision for me; but I believe the pain has some purpose, much like that experienced during childbirth."
"Of course, not being a mother, I couldn't possibly comment on the pros and cons of labour pain!" said Niall.

Matthew's first battle with the grim reaper came sooner than he had anticipated. He got up for work as normal and started brushing his teeth as usual, in the bathroom. Suddenly, he experienced an enormous pain in his stomach, but this was no normal pain, for he promptly blacked out with little recollection of the series of events other than that when he came round, he was slumped in the bath, embarrassingly aware that he had soiled himself. However, he was thankfully still alive; nor was he left in some comatose state, but, interestingly, suddenly rendered hyper-aware. It was as if, as with Saul, scales had been removed from his eyes.

In his former existence, whether deliberately or not, his brain had filtered out anything it thought he could not cope with or should not see. Now the veil had been lifted and a new life began almost immediately. After only half an hour of enduring inertia, he was returned to the Earth with renewed vigour: perhaps this was ***vigour mortis***, he mused. What he resented, however, was the lack of control he had over that near-death experience. Next time, he thought, I want to be aware of every stage in the operation.

It was to be another decade before this opportunity arose.
"Why don't you take something for the pain?" Niall had suggested, "there's a whole new range of analgesics you could try."
"I wouldn't even take paracetamol," replied Matthew, "the pain's there for a purpose. It's warning me about something. If I can't feel it, I won't have any indication what might be wrong with me."

After quite a long journey driving down to Edinburgh, Matthew experienced, initially, some shoulder pain. After adjusting his seating position, he felt a slight tingling sensation in his fingers. All of this was just mildly annoying for him, but then a whole collection of indicators that all was not well emerged: the tightness across his chest was accompanied by a sensation in his throat that made him decide to pull over into a lay-by. He finally detected an unusual tingling sensation localised in an area on the top left hand side of his head. Similar symptoms reappeared just two days later, which, though worrying, he decided to ignore, and luckily for him, he returned to his reasonably fit state of health, resuming gentle exercise and modifying his diet towards the vegetarian end of the spectrum.

It was at this point that Jean-Paul reappeared to counsel him.
"Remember Matthew, that you rats, unlike cats, do not have nine lives. It's a case of three strokes and you're out; so don't go inviting trouble again. You've a lot to achieve before you die, but you do have just one more chance."
"I thought," said Matthew, "that everything was preordained: don't you already know the exact date and time of my death?" Jean-Paul reminded Matthew that free will had a part to play,
"You can cheat fate, if you really want to, you know," said Jean-Paul. "Even when one existence comes to an abrupt end, that very event can trigger the start of a whole new life, if you so desire."

Matthew wondered what such a transmigration of his soul would entail,
"How would I know I was really alive again and not just some lingering set of after-images or persistent memories reincarnated into some zombie form?" Jean-Paul smiled.
"Believe me, Matthew; you'll know ***metempsychosis*** when it hits you!" Matthew was apprehensive,
"Does that mean my spirit might be reincarnated in the body of a rat?" he asked. Jean-Paul hesitated.
"It depends on how determined you are to make a difference in your next existence. If your resolve is weak, you might well come back as a donkey; but if you truly care enough to challenge world leaders about their stewardship of the Earth, you'll be happy to know that something approaching human form is your most likely transfiguration."

The next thing he knew, Matthew was undergoing an out-of-body experience, looking at his physical form in a totally detached kind of way. It was how he remembered being hypnotised at the dentist's to numb practically all sensation of pain. As the doctors prodded and poked his recumbent torso, he observed the body's reactions with a rather limited degree of attention. Whether the medics took blood samples, intubated or applied the paddles to defibrillate, his soul just looked on in a ***disinterested*** kind of way.

Matthew did not so much worry what would happen to his body when he died: it was his soul that he wanted to preserve. But first of all, he had a number of outstanding matters he wanted settled before his departure.

## Chapter seventy-two – the funeral director

***All the world's a stage,***
***And all the men and women merely players:***
***They have their exits and their entrances***

***Shakespeare – As you like it***

As an actor, Matthew had learnt that it was vitally important to be able to take direction, but he was damned if he was going to have his one and only exit stage-managed by a funeral director; especially one who had adopted the catchy phrase, ***mind how you go!*** taken from the salutation of the old-fashioned bobby on the beat, but modified it by the substitution of the exclamation mark for a question mark for use in his promotion materials. ["Mind how you go?"] As an earth rat, Matthew was inclined to favour burial; but he also liked the idea of rising from the ashes like a phoenix after cremation. But then he recalled an ominous remark:
"When you die, I'm going to dance on your grave!" Matthew's bitter enemy, Ivan, had threatened.
"That's settled it, then," said Matthew. "I'm going to ask to be buried at sea!"

Matthew had a word with, George, the undertaker, just to set the record straight,
"I'd like you to be more of a master of ceremonies, if you don't mind. I've always found these occasions far too stuffy, solemn and formal." The undertaker protested, "But that's how they're meant to be, funerals. People have to be encouraged to show some respect for the dear departed." Matthew's thoughts promptly strayed to the tasty venison the band had enjoyed after the night Niall had driven into a stag.
"To the deer departed!" came the toast, as they quaffed their champagne. Only a penetrating stare from the undertaker brought him back to Earth with a jolt.

"Oh, sorry," said Matthew, "I was about to tell you how I wanted my funeral conducted. Now, to start with, I want loud lively music to accompany my departure – preferably live music to compensate for a dead musician. A local band playing Queen's ***Bohemian Rhapsody***, perhaps, or ***Interstellar Overdrive*** by Pink Floyd." George frowned,
"that will present quite a challenge; but I'll see what I can do," he mumbled.

"Then there's the flowers," said Matthew. "I don't want chrysanthemums under any circumstances. And not orchids[42]: etymologically speaking, they're just a load of bollocks! No, for a gladiator like myself, only gladioli[43] will do."
"What about the readings," said the undertaker, "have you any preference as to what texts you would like?" Matthew chewed over a perplexing variety of options in that area, before arriving at a most appropriate choice.
"Dulce et decorum est pro patria mori.[44]"
"Cause of death?" asked the registrar.
"I shall die for my country," came the reply from Matthew, "we all have to look for a justification for dying, just as much as we might seek a reason for living."

"And now – how can I address this rather delicate matter – after you have been dispatched, how would you like the wake to proceed?" inquired George. Matthew recalled an old Frank Carson joke, where a couple of guests invited to the wake were somewhat the worse for wear after imbibing liberally all day. As they supported themselves against the piano which had its lid open, one turned to the other and asked, in his intoxicated state,
"Who was he, then?" The other equally intoxicated guest replied, looking down at the piano,
"Oi've no idea, but didn't he have a lovely set of teeth?"
"Plenty of booze," said Matthew, "and lots of unhealthy food. Let the mourners drown their sorrows and 'let them eat cake'. In my experience, people like to compensate for the loss of a loved one (or even a not-so-loved one) with a little cupboard love."

"What about the eulogy?" asked the undertaker. Matthew had, in his time, written a few of these and read them out for friends, so he was hoping that his own would follow a similar structure. The historian within him had always tried to identify significant dates in history with the age and status of the deceased, along with any impact that some world event might have had on the individual.
"My mother, for example," Matthew began, "was born in 1905. She would have been aged seven when the Titanic went down; eleven when the Great War broke out. Her adolescence would have coincided with the Roaring Twenties and with the widespread availability to the masses of the so-called Crystal Set, designed to receive radio broadcasts, at minimal cost to the listener."

Matthew looked for further major events in the twentieth century.

---

[42] "testicle"
[43] "little swords"
[44] Horace / Wilfred Owen

"By the time World War Two broke out, my mother was thirty-four and still single; but she married my father exactly half-way through the war, when he was home on leave whilst serving in North Africa and Italy." George suddenly became animated,
"So you must have been amongst those born to mothers in their forties, like I was myself. I don't know how you found that experience yourself – for me it was okay, because I was an only child and spoilt something rotten. You know how grandparents tend to do that nowadays? Well, I felt increasingly that my parents were starting to slip into aged grandparent mode." Matthew had had a similar experience,
"But my parents always made up for their lack of energy by making sure I felt loved," he said.

Matthew returned to his own personal eulogy,
"I was born in 1948, the year that the Olympic Games were held in London. Other significant dates for me were: 1969 (aged twenty-one) when I spent a year in Germany and coincidentally when Neil Armstrong ***allegedly*** walked on the moon; twenty years later, in 1989, I was again in Germany; this time to witness the demolition of the Berlin Wall. The Orwellian year of 1984 had passed without incident and the dreaded Y2K melt-down only delivered limited collateral damage when I reluctantly elected to go on a retreat to a "croft for the crazy", or, in the English vernacular, a funny farm.

"2001 was marked by my rehabilitation into that particular rat race that is supposed to constitute normality, and coincided, of course, with the destruction of the twin towers. I watched Jim's computer screen in horror as the planes hit: Jim was an American colleague, and I watched as he stared at the pictures in total disbelief. I felt great empathy with Jim at that point: it could just as easily have been the UK on the receiving end." George, himself - one might reasonably assume - almost inured to death, was clearly upset, too.
"Such an enormous loss of lives," he commented. Then he got Matthew to continue his plans for the eulogy,
"And 2012: what happened in that year?"

Matthew thought it quite apt to be aged sixty-four when the London Olympics came around again,
"Well, at least Nostradamus' promised Armageddon didn't materialise," said Matthew. "And, I must admit, I was happy to be able to spend some time with my grandchildren and see them grow up; who'd have expected Luke to become an astronaut, or Leni a submariner, for that matter?" The undertaker had one last question,
"Did you expect to survive until 2025," he asked. Matthew smiled,
"I can't honestly say I expected ***the planet*** to survive that long in its present form: I never imagined mankind being able to adjust to such a rapid reversal in the polarity of the Earth."

George had been impressed by the ability of world powers to finally realise that their individual survival depended upon mutual cooperation.
"Instead of blocking immigration, as I thought they quite understandably would, once precious resources became scarce, they began to actively encourage the mass migration of nations. What had once been lands flowing with milk and honey, like Canaan, had now become either frozen wastes or arid deserts; on the other hand, whole new areas of verdant pastures and luscious vegetation had sprung up in previously uninhabitable areas of the world.

"The trick was to reorganise the peoples of the world, encouraging them to find a new life in the settlements. The previously affluent countries of the northern hemisphere were turned overnight into impoverished beggars." Matthew remembered the generous reaction of the southern hemisphere,
"They could have just said, 'now see how you like it for a change!' but they were sufficiently magnanimous to offer their assistance to the North. Of course," added Matthew wryly, "the more tolerant you are of chaos, the more adaptable you can be when the unexpected happens. We bipolars are ideally suited to adapting to the sudden change!" The undertaker was not without a sense of humour,
"That would account for the survival of the bipolar bears, too, I suppose? Now, where is your next port of call?"

"I'm just off to check my facts with Veronica, the librarian," said Matthew.

**Chapter seventy-three – the archivist**

"1948 – It seems like an eternity ago, doesn't it?" remarked Matthew. Veronica, the librarian, agreed,
"As soon as we entered the twenty-first century, I started to feel old, because when I got the new forms to complete, instead of inserting my date of birth as 03/09/48, I now had to start adding the '19'. Veronica, like all librarians Matthew had ever met, had always been extremely helpful, so when he asked her to help him research the year when they were both born, he knew she would come up trumps.

Veronica suffered chronic pain, but like most of those who experience genuinely agonizing pain, she never complained. The pain revealed itself – to those who cared enough to notice – in her permanent kyphosis, since this condition lead to her walking with a stoop. She always met the customers with a smile, and never so much as raised her voice to them, despite their irritating habit of expecting her to drop every other task she might be engaged in, in order to render immediate assistance to them, as if life itself depended on it.

"Let's narrow down the search first of all," she suggested. "Knowing your penchant for music, shall we start there?" Matthew thought that this was an excellent place to start. He imagined the tunes, both popular and classical, his parents would have been listening to on their primitive radio apparatus. He remembered a huge monstrosity of a radio, attached to an 'accumulator'. The latter appeared to work on the same principal as a car battery and would require regular topping up with sulphuric acid and distilled water. The aerial went on for what seemed to the young Matthew like miles around the house. Despite all this paraphernalia, the signal came and went quite erratically, with the result that you never heard a complete song all the way through. Matthew imagined, whilst still in the womb, hearing these sounds which occasionally approached a quality worth listening to, provided that the so-called 'sweet spot' had been found for the direction the aerial had to point.

"So would you like to know who they might have been listening to?" asked Veronica. "Yes please," said Matthew.
"It seems most likely, on the classical side, that Shostakovich and Stravinsky would have predominated that year," said Veronica.
"A bit too heavy for my parents, I would think," said Matthew, "I seem to remember tenor voices, like Richard Tauber." Veronica jogged his memory,
"How about one called 'Love's old sweet song'? she suggested. Matthew was astounded. The song came back to him as if it were yesterday. He could not resist singing it aloud,

"Just a song at twilight, when the lights are low, and the flickering shadows softly come and go... - That was my grandmother's, (Rosa's) favorite song," said Matthew. "1948 was also the year of Richard Tauber's death," added Veronica.

"I remember the tunes of some fantastic composers proliferating around that time, too," said Matthew.
"Cole Porter and Irving Berlin composed some delightful tunes," said Veronica, "and of course there were lots of musicals and films around that year." Matthew remembered his mother repeating lines from the Wizard of Oz, such as: 'come out, come out, wherever you are!'
"Who would have imagined back then," he said to Veronica, "that homosexuality would eventually be legalized, with ***Friends of Dorothy*** being openly gay and revealing their affection for Judy Garland?"

"Did your parents possess a gramophone?" asked Veronica.
"No," said Matthew, "not until we moved house in the 1950's: it was one you had to wind up, and change the needle each time you put on another record. We did, however, eventually get a ***Dansette*** model that would play 45's and thirty-three-and-a-third, as well as 78's."
"You might be interested to know that Columbia produced the first long-playing record in 1948," said Veronica, "it meant that you could hear about half-an-hour's worth of songs before you had to turn it over."
"Before you ask, Veronica," said Matthew, "my parents never had a phone, either: in emergencies we would go out to the public call-box with four old pennies, and if we didn't make a connection, we pressed button 'B' to get our money back. Making a phone call was then deemed to be the very pinnacle of technological ability – so much so, that I actually got a special badge in the Scouts for successfully contacting Arkala." Veronica smiled,
"I trust you did your best?" she said, remembering the 'dyb, dyb, dyb' motto of the scouts.

"Let's look at all those advances in social provision after the war," suggested Matthew.
"Where do you want to start?" asked Veronica, recalling the plethora of legislation that was introduced that year.
"NHS – good or bad idea?" asked Matthew.
"Well," said Veronica, "you should remember that prior to the NHS, only the reasonably well-off could afford the charges made by doctors, dentists and the like, so it was introduced as a necessary safety-net. We tend to take it all very much for granted nowadays."
"But it's increasingly getting privatized again by stealth," said Matthew.
"Just be patient," said Veronica. "Maybe it will go the way of the trains."
"How do you mean?" asked Matthew.
"Well, in 1948, the railways were nationalized, though if you remember, the carriages still had first, second and third class compartments. They were

privatized again in the 1980's. But the desire for nationalization will probably return eventually: look what's started to happen to the banks!"

"And I've got down here 'national assistance', whatever was that?" asked Matthew. "A benefits system, originally created to provide for a small group of very needy individuals to help them survive," said Veronica. "Of course, it's been abused over recent years: only North Sea Oil kept it afloat." Matthew nodded.
"I'm now seeing three generations of families who've never had to work for a living – surely that wasn't the original intention?" Veronica did not say a word, but the expression on her face told him all he wanted to know.

Veronica now moved on to inventions around at the time.
"You probably wouldn't have realized that ***Velcro*** was invented in 1948, would you?" she asked.
"Not really something I'd be interested in," said Matthew.
"So what about technical advances?" asked Veronica.
"I think I remember reading about 1948 being the year the first ever computer was developed – in Manchester, wasn't it?" said Matthew.
"Yes," said Veronica, "Freddie Williams and his team pioneered that invention."
"We've certainly come a long way since then," said Matthew, observing his palm-held computer, "Their computer was basically mechanical and took up the space of an entire room."

"Do you recall the world leaders of the day?" asked Veronica.
"Joseph Stalin always comes to mind, for some reason," replied Matthew.
"Probably because of the Berlin airlift," said Veronica, "the Russians tried to blockade Berlin, but the allies kept the Berliners supplied with food and other essentials by making drops from aeroplanes. And do you know which country was created in 1948?" asked Veronica.
"Wasn't it Israel?" guessed Matthew.
"Yes," replied Veronica, "and do you remember Gandhi?"
"Yes, of course," said Matthew.
"Well," said Veronica, "he was assassinated in 1948." Matthew thanked Veronica for providing such detailed information.
"See you later," said Veronica, "oh, and give my regards to Charon."

Matthew found the whole exercise of contextualizing his arrival on this Earth immensely fulfilling. He felt that now he could take his place in history, whether as a minor celebrity or just as a footnote. But how would he be able to contextualize his departure?

## Chapter seventy-four – the ferryman

"Come with me," said Jean-Paul, in his newly-revealed role of psychopomp, "I'll give you a guided tour of the underworld."
"Where exactly ***is*** that?" asked Matthew, feeling some small but not insignificant degree of trepidation about such an impending journey.
"I used to think it was other people, but now I realise it's probably best seen as a voyage into the unconscious."
"I notice," said Matthew, "that you regard it as a voyage: that would suggest a boat-trip, I assume?"
"Not in my language," said Jean-Paul, "but, as it happens, you're right to make that assumption. Oh, and by the way, you'll need one of these," he said handing Matthew an old penny.

"Can't I pay with decimal currency?" Matthew asked. Jean-Paul explained, "Charon still trades in libra and denarii." Matthew remembered a time when the currency was pounds, shillings and pence.
"Doesn't he take shillings, too?" Jean-Paul shook his head.
"They don't like division[45] here, much: look where Mohammed and Ali ended up." Matthew recalled Dante's view that they belonged in a region of hell only one circle removed from the devil. He felt this was unjust,
"Surely they were both good men: what was their great crime in Dante's eyes?" Jean-Paul sighed,
"Disunity. Schism. It was thought that all breakaway faiths sowed the seeds for future conflict."

Matthew reflected:
"But they weren't exactly an all-embracing faith themselves, were they, the Christians?" Jean-Paul agreed, to a certain extent,
"Dante put Saladin in the first level, Limbo, amongst those who were virtuous souls despite not being Christians." Matthew turned next to the Jewish faith,
"And why do you think usury comes out as such a heinous sin?" he asked, "Only one level below the sowers of discord, the false prophets."
"I must admit," said Jean-Paul, "that a certain degree of anti-Semitism might have been prevalent in the Florence of the fourteenth century, so it is not inconceivable that Jewish money-lenders would have been reviled at the time and doomed to the delights of level seven, along with blasphemers, sodomists and politicians." Matthew looked Jean-Paul straight in the eye, "You'll have to watch out for yourself, too: ***mentors*** are located there, too!"

"Look at this picture!" said Jean-Paul. Böcklin's painting of the English cemetery with its funereal cypress trees at the start of their journey

[45] Etymology of shilling suggests splitting process

reminded Matthew of his own trip to Florence. In the Anglican Church, he had joined an operatic tenor in the chorus of ***O sole mio***.
"Now look again," said Jean-Paul, "There's Psyche!" Matthew felt sorry for the poor soul,
"Love can be very cruel," he said, "But where's Cupid?" Jean-Paul smiled,
"Off on some erotic adventure, no doubt," he said. "Now let's get Phlegyas to navigate us along the subterranean streams of your subconscious mind."

In witnessing his own demise, Matthew experienced most of the emotions manifested after the death of a loved one, as he travelled down the five rivers: sorrow and tears, of course, but also feelings of denial – why did this have to happen to him, just when he was about to be successful in life. He experienced anger and hatred in equal measure as he passed through the river of boiling blood and on to the river Styx.
"A trip down memory lane next – or was that forgetfulness?" said Jean-Paul. "You know how the false prophets were condemned to see only behind them as a punishment for pretending to predict the future?" he said. Matthew nodded. "Did you ever wonder about going senile – you know, suffering from dementia?" Matthew admitted that it had concerned him, because he was frequently losing brief interludes of time.
"Sometimes, when I was playing in the band, it happened: and I found myself confusing things, as well as forgetting what I'd originally set out to do."

Jean-Paul elaborated his thesis:
"Like those in hell who tried to predict the future, you condemned yourself to thinking backwards. You'd remember vividly some event that happened over fifty years ago, but you'd have forgotten something that had only just happened. You'd escaped into in a fantasy world of the Golden Age, where life was so much better – in theory – because you found the modern world with all its technological advances far too scary to contemplate. Now, if you want to preserve your marbles, start living in the present and continue planning for the future."

Matthew watched as they reached a confluence: he had to choose Lethe or Mnemosyne. Fortunately for him, he opted for the latter: a waking dream kept him alert.
"How long will this journey take?" he asked. Jean-Paul gave a frank response,
"At least four months," he said, "rebirth, like nature herself, comes in the spring – just ask Persephone. She still hibernates down here with her husband for a third of the year."

Matthew wanted to ask Jean-Paul's view of the perplexing variety of options concerning what to do with your body after death.
"What would you recommend?" asked Matthew.

"They say cryogenics is the modern way to go," said Jean-Paul, "But you wouldn't want to end up like Judas, encased in ice on level nine, now would you? You might like to ask Phoenix over there: he's a big fan of cremation. And burial? Personally, I don't like the idea of vicarious cannibalism suggested in the song, ***On Ilkley Moor Baht 'At***. But then, why are you bothered about your bag of bones at all? It's your soul you should be looking after. Remember what I told you: ***be yourself!***"

"Am I not allowed an ***alter ego***; the persona I choose to display to the world?" said Matthew.
"Beware of being two-faced," warned Jean-Paul, "Remember where the hypocrites ended up!" Matthew checked his guide-book,
"Level eight," he said. Does everyone get their come-uppance in the hereafter?"
"I think you'll find that punishment is often meted out long before the hereafter," said Jean-Paul.
"That's just ***karma***," said Matthew, "But tell me, would you not agree that every individual has to be a composite?"

Jean-Paul shrewdly counselled against the fragmentation process, but highlighted some distinct elements.
"Matthew," he said, "I take it you're now comfortable with your feminine side, your ***anima***?" Matthew nodded.
"I can appreciate her intuitive nature," he said.
"And your shadow, do you acknowledge that?" asked Jean Paul.
"I take it you're referring to my dark side. I now feel I have utterly embraced that part of myself with impunity: he's a vital component of my new personality."

"Time to step aboard the roundabout," said Jean-Paul.
"But it's spinning too fast for us to get on," said Matthew.
"That's because we're just outside limbo," said Jean-Paul, "If we board at a level closer the centre, it will be moving much more slowly, and we'll be able to hop on board. I suggest level six – you might like to see what can happen to hedonists like yourself." Matthew protested,
"***carpe diem***: that was my motto. I never went for all that self-denial that those stiff-upper-lip Stoics advocate. After all, ***Cui bono***[46]?"

Jean-Paul showed him how easy it was, now that they had joined the merry-go-round, to proceed to the adjacent level which accommodated suicides.
"What are they doing?" asked Matthew.
"They're eternally condemned to self-harm," said Jean-Paul, "It's the only way they can gain relief from pain."

---

[46] Who benefits (from that)?

"Next level, please!" said Matthew, fascinated at whom he might find on level eight. "Along with the pimps," said Jean-Paul, "you'll find the flatterers. They must be one of your favourite groups of people." Matthew was puzzled,
"How come?" asked Matthew.
"They spent their lives talking crap. Not a genuine remark ever," said Jean-Paul.
"I take it they were sentenced to be subjected to defecation from on high into eternity?" asked Matthew, knowing that the punishment had to fit the crime.

"Then there's the folk who tried to trade in the things that money cannot buy," said Jean-Paul.
"I've just spotted a famous politician," said Matthew, "what was Simon's crime?" Jean-Paul explained,
"He thought he could buy ministerial office. They're just like drug- and people-traffickers. They think that money will buy them anything they want." Matthew suddenly noticed a lizard, slithering off into the distance,
"Who was he?" he asked. Jean-Paul explained,
"Thieves are condemned to become reptiles." Matthew spotted a toad,
"why's he got eggs attached to his hind legs?" he asked. "Nothing sinister there," said Jean-Paul, "He's a midwife- toad. You'll occasionally hear him croaking the song, ***Stand by your woman!***"

## Chapter seventy-five – the neonate

"Now you remember how to regress, don't you?" asked Jean-Paul.
"You mean that thing we used to do under hypnosis?" replied Matthew. Jean-Paul agreed.
"Though you never tried to access your previous existences, I take it?" Matthew had taken his volunteers back as far as their childhood, noting how their behaviour mirrored the abilities and attitudes of individuals at key stages in their development. Jean-Paul wanted to know if Matthew had taken them back to being a baby,
"Did you try out the Babinski Reflex?" he asked. Matthew nodded,
"The one where you run a pencil down the sole of the foot?" Jean-Paul was curious, "And did the hypnotically regressed adult respond in the anticipated manner?" Matthew could not honestly say that the way the toes fanned out was convincing proof of actual regression, though he had successfully regressed adults to childhood and asked them to draw pictures. The latter were clearly at the level of a child.
"The results were – shall we say – somewhat ambiguous," said Matthew.
"Well, this time you'll be able to gain access to former lives: I take it you're comfortable with the notion of self-hypnosis?" Matthew reflected.
"Isn't all hypnosis really self-hypnosis? After all, the subject has to be a willing accomplice for it to work, at least in my experience. I'm not really taken in by all that Svengaliesque hypnotic power." Jean-Paul smiled.
"It's surprising how effective theatricality can be," he said. "Now remember to keep this knowledge secret. If you start claiming you can communicate with the spirit world, they'll have you locked up again. Conduct your séances in total privacy so that no one can listen in on your dialogue with the dead. It will seem strange at first, especially when your new self starts to interrogate your old self, but you'll soon get used to it. Now, are you ready for the funfair? Here comes the flume!" Suddenly, Matthew was on his own again, heading down what he later realized had been the birth canal towards the light.
"Hello, little fellow!" said Persephone, the midwife, cleaning him up and handing him to his mother.

The question was: did he really need to repeat all his childhood years? After all, he had already inherited the collective wisdom of generations that preceded him. He decided to skip school, and resume life aged twenty, at that crucial stage when you have to find a job and get married. This time he chose a creative profession that encompassed music, drama and photography, but he became impatient to see where his new life was heading.
"Observe the life-line on your left hand," the clairvoyant had said, "that's your potential life-expectancy, slightly better than three score years and

ten." Matthew had been reasonably content with that prediction, but he had wondered what his right hand had to say.
"Now compare that line with the corresponding line on your right hand," said the clairvoyant. "As you see, the continuity is interrupted and I would venture to suggest that this matches the point in your life when you experienced a break-down." Matthew looked concerned,
"Does that suggest a near-death experience?" The clairvoyant was doubtful,
"Not necessarily," she said.
"How do I read the continuation of my life-line?" asked Matthew.
"Imagine you have a rail network, and the track gets blocked after a land-slip. The train will have to be diverted around the blockage." Matthew could clearly see that new lines had been constructed to reconnect the previous link.

In Edinburgh, September 2008, Paolo, the media man, showed trainees how to spin their life stories. Matthew was particularly intrigued by the interview techniques shown in the training, partly because he had always fancied being a politician, and liked the fact that they somehow managed never to answer the question posed by the interviewer. Of course, from his time spent teaching media studies, he had already gleaned an insight into the vulnerability of spokespersons, not necessarily during the interview, but actually after the interview, when any film-editor worth his salt could rearrange clips to portray the very opposite message to that intended by the interviewee. The interviewer even had a trump card to play after the actual interview. He/she would generally re-record his/her set of questions – partly, it is true, to ensure that he or she could correct any obvious ***faux-pas*** or where lines had been fluffed; though, chiefly, at least in Matthew's experience, to manipulate the message by conducting a total re-write and re-recording of a whole new set of questions. It was then the team's job to ensure that the various sound-bites ***segued*** comfortably into one another.

Since Matthew had indicated his previous involvement with such techniques, Paolo explained how Matthew could apply a similar process to his new life.
"Imagine your life, not as a bowl of cherries, but as a compilation of videos that you can run, over and over again, if you like. You have sole control of the edit suite. You can fast forward, freeze time into a single frame, or you can even reverse the action if you so choose." Matthew found the analogy most appropriate.
"And, from a psychological point of view, I can erase undesirable memories. I can jettison the baggage, get rid of the crap," said Matthew. Paolo indicated another way that Matthew's new life could be re-written,
"You can even ***replace*** unpleasant memories with whole new scenarios," he said. "There is no script for you to learn and act out. You should establish a link to the message you want to go out to the world, as you do with the searching questions posed by a shrewd interviewer."

Paolo then presented Matthew with three huge boxes.
"In the first box," said Paolo, "you'll find a set of photo albums; in the second, rewritable DVD's; and in the third, a set of diaries. Would you like to take a look?" On inspection, the albums, disks and diaries were blank.
"It's very kind of you to present me with so many gifts, but if you don't mind me asking, why are they all blank? Wouldn't it have been a nicer touch to include some photos, footage or autobiographical text?" Paolo smiled,
"As I already told you, your new life is a ***tabula rasa***. It is up to you to compile the content."

Matthew recalled the children's TV presenter, Johnny Ball, once pointing out to kids that they were capable of achieving whatever they set their heart on; the greatest obstacle, he said, was their own self-doubt. That same lack of confidence had prevented Matthew from making sensible decisions in his former life. Though he would never have admitted it, Matthew was a bit of a perfectionist, and always thought others perceived him as a bit of a ***chancer***; a jack of all trades, maybe, but ultimately master of none.
"Even if you were a square peg in a round hole at times, you showed yourself capable of making a job your own, rewriting your job description as you went along," said Paolo. "Your main asset was your reliability – this can count for more than mere competence in most situations in life." It was true, Matthew did not like letting people down, and he would bust a gut to ensure he could make gigs with the band, even if his performance often left something to be desired.

One night at a regular venue, he had found himself introducing one of his self-penned songs as follows:
'And now a song I wrote some forty years ago, ***Take it while you can do***.' Deep inside, he still imagined himself as the nineteen-year-old, singing the song. But the lyrics suited a young adult, not a 'superannuated hippy', as ***Rita*** might have called him. Ironically, the lyrics seemed to have advocated a life-style that he never embraced himself – he was too much of a play-it-safe prevaricator to practise what he was preaching in the song.

Perhaps, in his efforts to be born again, he was already attempting to rewrite the story of his life. He donned a pair of sunglasses, psychologically indicating a need to restore his virginity. He wanted to un-break the glass in the windows of this dilapidated building that was himself.

## Chapter seventy-six – the glazier

In Matthew's day, one of the rites of passage for bored kids was to smash windows in derelict buildings. His mates clearly derived immense satisfaction out of the whole enterprise: not only because there was that unmistakably pleasing ***sound*** of breaking glass, but also because there was the adrenalin rush felt by the gang, knowing that the very noise generated might alert the powers-that-be to their crime. But for Matthew, the fixer, it seemed such a destructive operation; he would have much preferred to be able to reverse the whole fragmentation process, and return the building to its pristine state.

"We don't just torment the souls, down here, you know," said Charon, "we also patch them up, ready for recycling. It all started as a cottage industry, but now it's an enterprise on an infernal scale." Matthew was fascinated.
"How is it done?" he enquired, "How do you put Humpty Dumpty back together again?" Charon showed Matthew the production line.
"First of all, we carefully place the fragments into the cauldrons. As with glass, people's souls need to be heated up to anything from 500 degrees Celsius to 3000 degrees, depending on the proportion of impurities in each individual soul."
"I see," said Matthew, "that would explain the need for fire down here; but I've also seen black hail; snow and ice, too – especially when we approached level nine." Charon asked Matthew to be patient,
"I was coming to that," he said. "The molten soul-mix is then poured into pre-constructed moulds, and rapidly cooled so that the restored soul can return to Earth, purged of former imperfections." Matthew noticed a group of workers equipped with what looked like enormous spoons,
"What are they doing?" he asked. Charon reminded Matthew that, down in the underworld, the punishment had to fit the crime.
"They were the trouble-makers, the stirrers, if you like, so it's quite appropriate, don't you think, that they have to keep stirring the mixture to ensure the elimination of bubbles? If bubbles weren't properly removed, some reconstructed souls could return full of hot air – hardly the productive individuals that we take such a pride in manufacturing here!"

"What happens," said Matthew, "if some fragments are missing?" thinking back to his earlier trade with the devil.
"No problem," said Charon, reassuringly. "We just activate the synecdoche machine."
"Pardon my ignorance," said Matthew, "but what exactly does that do?"
"Pars pro toto[47]" replied Charon, "Or, in other words, to satisfy the scientist within you, it's like stem cells: they don't just have a multipotential in their

[47] The part represents the whole

applications, particularly the embryonic ones – they, like God, are omnipotent." Matthew still did not quite get it,
"I really don't understand the science you're alluding to."

"That pane of glass you and your mates broke all those years ago: how do you imagine the glazier knew what type and pattern it was?"
"I assume," said Matthew, "that he got that information from one of the broken fragments."
"Correct," said Charon, "and it's just like with DNA: each fragment of your soul contains the blueprint for your reconstruction, so any missing pieces don't ruin the final appearance of the completed jigsaw-puzzle." Matthew wondered what happened to the crap elements of his soul, now that he had offloaded them onto the devil. "Lucifer is happy to double as a garbage collector. He provides this service to ensure that mankind can evolve. If mankind had stuck to routine over the millennia, we'd still be living in the Stone Age." Matthew was curious,
"So what happens to the garbage?"
"It gets recycled," said Charon, "one man's crap is another man's archaeological evidence. How do you think we know so much about the diet of ancient man?"

It was at this point that Jean-Paul rejoined Matthew just to inform him what had happened to all his assassinated characters and the memories with unpleasant connotations. They had been frozen in time as photographic images. Some early memories would appear to be sepia; later memories would appear as black-and-white or more recent memories in glorious Technicolor, as they used to say.

## Chapter seventy-seven – the curator

"All your characters have been ***freeze-framed*** in the Rogues' Gallery," said Jean-Paul. "I suggest you get Veronica, the new curator, to show you around." After this brief introduction, Jean-Paul was gone. Matthew already knew that many of his ***personae*** were archetypical figures that often visit us in our dreams. As we know, he liked the idea, suggested to him by his wife, Anita, of framing traumatic events before locking them away in an imaginary gallery of photographs for future reference, if absolutely necessary. Memories, he believed, should never be erased, because they are part of our identity and we should learn from traumatic experiences, whilst at the same time never allowing them to control our thinking.

"Hello, again, Matthew," said Veronica. "You'll be wanting the guided tour of the Rogues' Gallery, I take it?" Matthew smiled,
"Yes, I'd rather like that, even though I am, of course, only too familiar with the villains." Veronica pointed out that despite its name, the gallery displayed some heroes, too,
"There's a fair mix of characters, some more salubrious than others," she said. Maybe I should have hung on to more of those, with their 'health-giving' properties, Matthew thought. Veronica first explained the layout of the gallery, handing Matthew a leaflet.

Matthew studied the leaflet meticulously.
"It seems very familiar," he said. Veronica explained that the famous female architect, Sarah Hussein, had wanted to get away from rectangular constructions generally favoured by male architects and so had modelled her designs on the more naturally occurring rounded shapes, based on human organs. This particular design appealed to Matthew, the designer, who had always wanted to create a sphere, as we may recall. Here it was, complete with left and right hemispheres.
"There are six chambers altogether, identified by specific function," said Veronica. "Can you still ride a bike, by the way?" Matthew found this a rather strange question, "Yes, of course I can; anyway, I thought skills once perfected couldn't effectively be 'unlearned'." Veronica suggested they start in the room on the left labelled ***putamen***, "This is where all the procedural memories are stored," she said.

"I recognise that guy," said Matthew, "that's the infamous musician – what's his name?" Veronica had to explain the system,
"Music represents a harmonious relationship between the inner self and life itself. You have to understand, Matthew, that none of these characters is ever named. That musical guy's a monotype." Matthew was confused,

"I've never heard of a monotype," he said. "Couldn't he at least be a ***stereotype***, given his musical background?" Taking this as a rhetorical question, Veronica moved on to her next exhibit.
"Do you recognise the artist?" she asked. "Looks rather like Adolf Hitler," said Matthew.
"Frustrated artists often become dictators," said Veronica. Pausing briefly to look at other characters, such as the cyclist and the roofer, Matthew's eyes eventually settled on ***The Cook***.
"Of all the people I met down there in my subconscious mind, he was the one person who offered the best explanation of the process of defragmentation," said Matthew.

"Let's move on to the next chamber – the one over there on the right," suggested Veronica. Matthew read the legend above the door, ***prefrontal cortex***.
"Funny name for a room," he commented.
"Eminently forgettable, if you're prone to dementia," said Veronica. "Actually, we shouldn't really have many specimens in here, because you need them for your day-to-day survival." Matthew suddenly spotted a familiar face,
"Who's that?" he asked.
"I'm sorry to have to tell you this, Matthew, but that one's ***The Communicator***. You've been displaying some difficulties recently in that department, I understand?" Matthew shook his head.
"Shall we move on to the ***cortex***?" suggested Veronica, "it might help you recall your various 'episodes'." Matthew was fascinated.
"There's ***The Taxi-driver***," he said.
"And don't forget ***The Teacher***," said Veronica, but Matthew was not interested, "Too many bad experiences," he said. "You should focus more on all the success stories," said Veronica, "you'd be surprised how many appreciative students you have out there."

"Look at the next big chamber, Matthew," said Veronica. Matthew read the legend, ***temporal lobe***.
"What's that?" asked Matthew.
"Precisely that!" replied Veronica, reflecting on all the factual content and attention to detail deposited there (i.e. ***what?***)
"There's ***The Etymologist***, and over there is ***The Economist***," said Matthew, but in the end, I suppose it's all just a thesaurus of useless information?" Veronica disagreed,
"Extensive factual knowledge is essential, if you want to draw on wisdom from a variety of subject areas. Intensive study of a limited number of disciplines can lead to convergent thinking, which is useless when you need to think out of the box. Now, if you would, turn right, and enter the ***amygdala*** room - we call it the 'F' room.

"Why's that?" asked Matthew.
"Fears, phobias and facial recognition," said Veronica.
"There's ***The Axe Man***," said Matthew, "and here's ***The Judge***; but who's that, I can't quite make him out." Veronica laughed,
"Can't you see? It's a looking glass." Matthew faced up to his mirror image, and was horrified to see the title of the exhibit, ***The Critic***.
"Let's move on, please, Veronica" he pleaded.

The final room was the ***hippocampus***, and true to form, Matthew quickly lost his bearings.
"Your kinaesthetic abilities seem to have let you down," said Veronica.
"Yes," said Matthew, "I've always had problems with spatial awareness – I'm no good at navigating whatsoever. That's why I appreciate ***satnav*** so much." Veronica offered a possible explanation for Matthew's disorientation,
"For you, Matthew, the twin concepts of time and place are conflated. The 'here and now' is still seriously undermined by the 'there and then'. In your waking life, the concept of ***time*** predominates; whereas, in your dreams, it is relative locations in ***space*** that represent the past, present and future."

"Any more exhibitions?" asked Matthew.
"There is one, but it's not normally available to the general public. We could, of course, make an exception in your case." Matthew was keen to investigate,
"Sounds more like an ***in***hibition, to me!" he said.
"Quite an astute comment, in the circumstances," said Veronica, "Come with me." Matthew followed her to a darkly-lit recess.
"There's Eve!" said Matthew,
"That's what I meant about losing your inhibitions!" said Veronica. Matthew noted the title, ***The Siren***.
"Press the button," said Veronica.
"Gosh, it's interactive!" said Matthew, watching as the portrait revolved to reveal ***The Anima*** on its reverse side. Further along, the devil was identified, not as Mephistopheles, but as ***The Shadow*** with the role of ***The Facilitator*** on the reverse.

Kate was at once ***The Princess*** and ***The Amazon***. Alice was clearly identifiable as ***The Kindly Mother*** alternating with ***The Competitor.***
"Who is this character?" asked Matthew.
"The one entitled ***The Villain***, you mean?" asked Veronica, "It depends on your mood, I suppose." Matthew was puzzled,
"What do you mean?" he said.
"Well," said Veronica, "Ivan the Terrible is the villain, but if you press the button, whom do you see?" Matthew pressed the button to reveal a familiar face.

"I thought ***I*** was supposed to be the critic," he said. "This looks like me again!" Veronica smiled.
"Maybe you're the angelic ***hero***, on this occasion."

Matthew rotated the image of ***The Journalist*** to reveal ***The Politician***. Veronica hazarded an explanation.
"They're both – at least in theory – supposed to be working for the greater public good." Matthew remained unconvinced of this fact.
"Look over there," said Veronica, "it's your old friend ***The Midwife Toad***. As you'll see, its very ugliness can be transformed into beauty through rebirth. There's a lesson for you, there, too. Then again, for you rats, whom others may perceive as disease-ridden vermin, there's power in the very excrement that the sewers convey." Matthew thought about his attempts to remove crap from his life.
"I think the manure symbolised my disintegration," he said. Matthew strayed over towards the inanimate objects. "I love ***The Kaleidoscope***. It's always fascinated me. I suppose it's like the way the defragmentation process used to be represented on the computer screen." Veronica smiled.
"So you haven't yet put away childish things?" she said, echoing the words of Saint Paul.

Next on his agenda was the image of ***The Nuclear Explosion***. Veronica, having once worked in the nuclear industry, was eminently qualified to offer an explanation. "You'll have heard of the phrase fission-fusion-fission, no doubt? It's rather like the creative process itself, isn't it? Disintegration and Dissent have to be replaced with Integration and Harmony. But then it starts all over again, just like the communist model." Matthew did not understand the analogy. "Revolution has to be ongoing to ensure the system doesn't atrophy," said Veronica.

"And here's a representation of ***The Parcel***," said Matthew, "Jean-Paul told me to keep its contents secret." Veronica suggested that this may be the wrong interpretation.
"The parcel represents your hidden talents," she said, "don't hide them under a bushel." Matthew next spotted ***The Puppeteer***. It was a complicated series of frames within frames.
"What's the significance of the frames?" asked Matthew. "It's to demonstrate to you that however much you feel in control, pulling the strings of all your marionettes that dance to your tune, there's always someone else pulling your strings, and they in turn, may be subject to the whims of an even higher authority." Matthew quoted his namesake.
"Watching us, watching them, watching you, I suppose?"

"What's ***The Shard of Glass*** signify?" asked Matthew.
"You've always been an outsider: Only when you have recognised your own fragmentation can you truly gain a sense of belonging," said Veronica.

"That picture over there looks interesting; I think I'll take a closer look," said Matthew. "Wait a minute – it's like seeing the world through glasses designed for someone else. The picture's totally distorted.
"We call that one ***The Wart***," said Veronica. "It represents, you'll be intrigued to know, distortion in our way of looking at the world." Matthew could not resist repeating his by now familiar acknowledgement, when attending ***Verrucas Anonymous***, "This is me, warts and all."

## Epilogue

The author is gratified to note the beginnings of some change in thinking in the psychiatric community. The reasons for this are complex; but suffice it to say that the recent UK government thinking behind moving away from purely pharmaceutical solutions to therapies such as ***mindfulness*** that encourage the patient to engage with thoughts and feelings seem quite promising. The reader will recall Matthew's recommendation to focus on the present, the ***here and now***; although he always had difficulty with the question words, ***where*** and ***when***: even at school geography and history were subjects that did not appeal to him, for some reason. Readers may have been put off, therefore, by the dearth of temporal and spatial signposts.

In order to embrace the moment, the author recommends keeping the mind engaged by undertaking creative, recreative and procreative activities. Such pursuits can stop the mentally ill from dwelling on traumatic events or failures that happened in the past which, as a consequence, dictate all the patient's anticipations of present and future experiences. The fascination with mental experiences, however bizarre or potentially hurtful, seems to have been - to some extent - his salvation, because, far from allowing the experiences to take control over his life, he decided to take an active part in controlling them. He was not prepared to become a passive victim of his experiences, but sought instead to understand them. Unlike many of his fellow- sufferers, who preferred to keep their experiences to themselves for fear of being ostracised by their community, he chose to be quite open about his breakdown, choosing instead to challenge a perceived universal stigma about mental ill-health. (We must beware of ***self-stigma***).

He does, however, have some difficulty with the advice offered in therapy to curb impulsive behaviour and replace it with 'conscious and deliberate' actions: Though he totally supports the notion of regaining control over your life by planning ahead, and hence not becoming dependent on others to make decisions for you, or relying on fate to determine your life experiences, he feels that the 'gut reaction' is one that really helps him to make decisions. Previously, he would have prevaricated and procrastinated so much that inactivity was the inevitable outcome. Equally, he believes that 'thinking about thinking' partially precipitated his breakdown, because that very self-analysis and reflection to the nth degree was so destructive, having, as it did, no synthesis or reconstruction to compensate for the disintegration it engendered. ***Metacognition*** needs handling with great care!

**Appendix (i) the deck of cards**

Mark = Four of Clubs (Responsibility)
Kate = Four of Hearts (Inspiration)
Matthew = Two of Spades (Gain)
Jean-Paul = Ace of Clubs (Spirituality)
Anita = Four of Diamonds (Charity)
Theodora = Three of Hearts (Opportunity)
Alice = Two of Diamonds (Loyalty)
Dr Sugar = Ace of Spades (Power)
Liam = Four of Spades (Freedom)
Liz = Queen of Hearts (Compassion)

## Appendix (ii) symbolic punctuation

**1.** [Alan]
**2.** [Alice]
**3.** [Anita]
**4.** "Bert"
**5.** Hazel?
**6.** [Helene]
**7.** Ivan !!!
**8.** Kate?
**9.** [Liam]
**10.** [Liz]
**11.** [Mark]
**12.** [Theodora]

***Key***: **[**safe**]**; **!** dangerous ; **"**what you see is what you get**"** **?** unknown quantity

**Bibliography**

Arcana Arcanorum, The Playing-Card Oracle, http://www.alcyone.com/aracana/oracle.html , date accessed: 07/07/2009

Ball, Pamela, 2003, *The Quantum Dream Dictionary*, London, Quantum

Bentall, Richard P., 2003, *Madness explained*, London, Penguin

Berk, Lesley, Berk, Michael, Castle, David & Lauder, Sue, 2008, *Living with Bipolar*, Sydney, Allen & Unwin

Böll, Heinrich, 1974, *Die verlorene Ehre der Katharina Blum*, Köln, Kiepenheuer & Witsch

Breggin, P.R., 1994, *Toxic Psychiatry*, St Martins Griffin

Cable, Vince, 2009, *The Storm*, London, Atlantic Books

Campbell, Alastair, 2008, *All in the Mind*, London, Hutchinson, Random House

Dürrenmatt, Friedrich, 1962, *Die Physiker*, Zürich, Verlags A.G. 'Die Arche'

Faulks, Sebastian, 2005, *Human Traces*, London, Hutchinson

Faulks, Sebastian, 2009, *A Week in December*, London, Hutchinson

Gillies, Andrea, 2009, *Keeper: Living with Nancy - a journey into Alzheimer's*, London, Short Books

Hamilton, Dr David R., 2008, *How your mind can heal your body*, London, Hay House

James, Oliver W, 2007, *Affluenza*, London, Vermillion

Kesey, Ken, 1962, *One flew over the Cuckoo's Nest*, New York, The Viking Press

Kirsch, Irving, 2009, *The Emperor's New Drugs, exploding the antidepressant Myth*, London, The Bodley Head

Kolb, David A., 1984, *Experiential Learning*, New Jersey, Prentice-Hall

Lynch, Terry, 2004, *Beyond Prozac*, Ross-on Wye, PCCS books.

Obama, Barack, 2006, *The Audacity of Hope*, New York, Random House

Peston, Robert, 2008, *Who runs Britain*, London, Hodder & Stoughton

Sawkins, John, 2008, *Rare Frequencies*, Brentwood, Essex, Chipmunkapublishing

Lightning Source UK Ltd.
Milton Keynes UK
UKOW01f0647140216

268280UK00001B/12/P